My sweetheart Chri...
for when I...
rub your head..... Mmmmm...!

♡ I love you sweetie

Your Love

♡

THE
Headache ♡
Book

Dr. Frank Minirth

with Sandy Dengler

A JANET
THOMA
BOOK

THOMAS NELSON PUBLISHERS
Nashville • Atlanta • London • Vancouver

Many thanks to Dr. Kevin Kinback, whose editing of the medical aspects of this book was invaluable.

Medical knowledge is constantly changing. Moreover, what may be true in the treatment of one individual may not apply to another. Therefore, the reader is encouraged to consult his/her local physician before applying any of the principles in this book.

Frank Minirth, M.D.

© 1994 by Frank Minirth, M.D. All rights reserved.

Written permission must be secured from the publisher to use or reproduce any part of this book, except for brief quotations in critical reviews or articles.

Published in Nashville, Tennessee, by Thomas Nelson, Inc., Publishers, and distributed in Canada by Word Communications, Ltd., Richmond, British Columbia, and in the United Kingdom by Word (UK), Ltd., Milton Keynes, England.

The information contained herein should not be relied upon for diagnosis or treatment for any illness, serious injury or disease and should not be used instead of seeking the services of a physician. A physician should be consulted immediately for treatment of any injury.

Unless otherwise indicated, Scripture quotations are from THE NEW KING JAMES VERSION of the Bible. Copyright © 1979, 1980, 1982, Thomas Nelson, Inc., Publishers.

Library of Congress Cataloging-in-Publication Information

Minirth, Frank B.
    The headache book / Frank Minirth, with Sandy Dengler.
      p.   cm.
    Originally published: Nashville: T. Nelson, 1994.
    Includes index.
    ISBN 0-7852-7715-3
    1. Headache—Popular works. I. Dengler, Sandy. II. Title.
RB128.M55 1995
616.8'491—dc20   94–46884
                                          CIP

Printed in the United States of America
4 5 6 7 — 99 98 97 96

Contents

CHAPTER 1

Misery

Your head throbs. Your temples pound. Your forehead feels like a gallon-sized melon squeezed into a quart jar. The ache behind your eye stabs so wickedly that you can't think. Distracted, harried by the relentless pain, you fumble for a couple more pills that will undoubtedly upset your stomach and may or may not alleviate your headache. Then you lie down, or wish to heaven you could, and pray that the misery will pass.

Or, a mild thudding sensation in your head alerts you to the fact that you have let the work, or the kids, or the exigencies of the moment get to you. You pop a couple of aspirin and continue with your day. But you're not as sharp as you ought to be, and you know it. Things slip through. You err. You miss little points and opportunities. Your headache hasn't stopped you, but it noticeably slows you down.

Every headache sufferer—and that includes nine of every ten adults and a surprising number of kids—has his or her own tale of woe, for headaches are as unique as the people who suffer from them. Headaches are our number one misery, not just now but throughout history.

Americans will spend half a billion dollars this year on over-the-counter pain remedies, most of which will be taken for headaches. Forty million Americans (that's one in every seven) will be disabled by headaches to the point of ceasing or curtailing daily activity. A recent survey of over ten thousand young people found that during a given month eight percent of the men and fourteen percent of the women would miss work or school because of headaches. It's worse when you're already sick. As I was making rounds at the hospital one morning, I asked how many had incapacitating headaches, a sort of straw vote. All fourteen patients raised their hands. Headaches can get in the way of other therapy, especially in a clinical, psychological setting. They distract. They replace more important issues.

Here at the Minirth Meier New Life Clinics, the typical person seeking help for headaches cries out, "My life is in ruins. These headaches are keeping me from functioning, and I can't get rid of them." The patient is not exaggerating. Headaches really are that debilitating for a lot of people, perhaps for you or for someone you know.

Joan arrived at my office a year ago, still in her bathrobe, her hair unkempt. Her husband, Mark, piloted her by the elbow to a chair and plopped down beside her.

"Dr. Minirth," the man opened, "this can't go on any longer. When one of Joan's migraines strikes, she's down flat for two days. She throws up; she can't move; she's miserable. Nothing seems to help. Look at her.

When she's okay, she's a powerhouse. She accomplishes so much. Right now I could draw more response out of a tree stump. I get a headache myself, just thinking about her. Is there any hope?"

Joan only said feebly, "I'm sorry you have to see me this way, Doctor."

Actually, I have seen patients in greater distress, but not many. She sat glassy-eyed and mopey, the picture of total hopelessness. I addressed her husband. "You made this appointment three months ago, Mark. How does it happen that Joan is in the midst of a migraine now, as you walk in the door?"

"I took a long shot—but not all that long a shot, I guess. They usually come around the time of her period. When I talked to your receptionist, I counted forward from her last period and made the appointment accordingly." Mark shrugged. "And we got lucky, so to speak."

So to speak. Joan would not have called it lucky, but it did help her situation. We were able to do a complete medical workup while she was actually experiencing her headache. We're not always able to do that.

The thorough medical evaluation is always the initial step in our treatment of severe headaches. The evaluation is not so much to discover causes as to rule out dangerous or life-threatening possibilities.

An example of the importance of this medical evaluation is the case of a youth worker who came to us with severe headaches. She had put on a hundred pounds as well. It had to be repressed anger, right? I was just out of school, and I knew these things. Well, we couldn't find any anger, but before long a surgeon removed a tumor the size of an orange from the frontal area of her brain.

When a headache strikes, particularly a kind of headache that has not happened before, the first thing the sufferer may think of is tumor or cancer or other dire possibilities. Dire possibilities become reality less than once in a hundred such cases. But we always want to rule out the possible life-threatening situations first. When we know what is not causing the headaches, we move on to exploring what is and then begin a treatment.

Remember that headaches are not a disease. They are a symptom of something else that is wrong. That something else can be *physiological* or *psychological*. If the cause is psychological, the headache is every bit as real as the one arising from physical causes. "It's all in your head" means nothing to the headache sufferer. Regardless of its origin, it still hurts.

To really appreciate how much it hurts, a person just about has to experience it. People who never get migraines seem certain that if the migraine sufferer would only take a pill and relax a few minutes, the headache would go away . . . as if the migraine sufferer (*migraineur*) were eagerly volunteering to undergo all this pain. People blessed with mild headaches or none at all tend to suspect victims of severe headaches of overdoing the complaints and moans. (Curiously, it usually doesn't work the other way; people who know severe headache pain firsthand do not often admire and praise people who complain of headache and carry on as if nothing were wrong.)

We at Minirth Meier New Life Clinics have seen excellent clinical success treating headaches, in large part because we tackle the problem aggressively and comprehensively. We know from experience that headaches are not a simple disorder you can treat with a pill and a pat on the back. They require a multi-pronged attack to heal body, mind, and spirit. Today, medicine has made such great gains in the treatment of headaches that it's ridiculous for people to suffer, let alone to continue functioning inadequately. Not only is a headache a complex thing with more than one root, there are also many diverse kinds of headaches.

The Many Faces of Headaches

"Excuse me, sir. Where are you from?"

"Why, I'm a European."

How many French, English, Italians, Spaniards, Swiss, or other Europeans would really respond with their continent instead of their nationality or even their regional origin? Wouldn't they answer instead, "I am a Catalonian, Señor" or "I am Sicilian"?

The term *headache* is the continent. The kinds of headaches are the nationalities. Although many share a common origin and some feel the same as others to their sufferers, they vary in scope, in degree of disablement, and in treatment. Joan was suffering a full-blown, devastating migraine. She was not over-dramatizing her discomfort; her headache really was draining her that badly.

Her husband, Mark, mentioned that he got a headache thinking about her. This pain was not just a sympathetic response. His was a tension headache. It was not debilitating, but it certainly was annoying. Same continent, different country. Joan's treatment and Mark's would vary greatly.

Figuring out what ails you isn't easy. Doctors even have trouble at times identifying the headaches they themselves suffer. However, knowing the several kinds of headaches and differentiating between them can help the layman in important ways. If you are not being seen by a doctor, you can get a better handle on what is happening inside your head. Perhaps a couple of aspirin are all you need. Perhaps you *should* see a doctor. We'll discuss the situations requiring medical intervention and the situations in which medical intervention would be helpful but not life-saving.

If you are already under a doctor's care, knowing about headaches will help you work better with your doctor in the management of your headaches. When you understand what your doctor is trying to do, you can cooperate better in the joint effort to master the monster, for it takes strong teamwork between doctor and patient to beat down a headache such as Joan's.

"Wait. Cooperate?" you say. "Of course I cooperate! I paid good money for my doctor's help. Why wouldn't I cooperate?"

Sadly, nearly half the patients we see do not. They change the timing or dosage of medicines or fail to take them at all. They always have a reason for their actions:

- "I felt better so I quit."
- "The medicine was too expensive to take all the time."
- "I found out my doctor prescribed an antidepressant, but I'm not depressed. Why should I be taking an antidepressant? Isn't that dangerous?"

- "I forgot to."
- "Our puppy chewed up the directions, so I just sort of took the pills like you would aspirin. Hey, it's just a headache, right?"

Such reasons can get colorful, but they are not medically valid. Different headaches coming from different origins require different kinds of medication—yes, even antidepressants, whether the patient is depressed or not. Dosages are customized for the person taking the medication. (That's why doctors warn you never ever to give your prescription to someone else, no matter how much their symptoms may resemble yours.)

We will get into some deep medical waters for several reasons. For one, doctors sometimes have trouble translating their medical language into explanations laymen can understand. We want to help with that, and at the clinic we find that our patients are remarkably interested in the more technical aspects of their problems and often show quite a bit of sophistication in their understanding. Even when we answer calls on our radio program, we frequently receive requests for technical information. I believe it is important that patients receive as much information as they can handle.

How Do You Spell Relief?

I trust, then, that this book will do several things for you besides show you where various kinds of headaches come from and how they differ:

- It will discuss medications and their effects in detail.

- It will discuss the life-style changes that are so often necessary for lasting relief.
- It will list seven steps all headache sufferers can use to help themselves.

In addition, I will offer help for dealing with headaches in children, things to do and things not to do. I will also discuss prevention, which is by far the better approach to treatment. Armed with that knowledge, you can approach the problem of your own headaches and those of your family members with far greater hope of finding a sound and lasting solution.

The bottom line, of course, is relief. Whether a headache is debilitating, like Joan's, or merely annoying, like Mark's, the sufferer yearns for relief.

And here I must offer an important word of caution. In perhaps one out of a hundred cases, a headache is the warning sign of a potentially dangerous condition. The brain needs plenty of oxygen all the time. In fact, deprived of oxygen for only a few minutes, adult brain cells begin to die. If the arteries feeding the brain clog up, rupture, or weaken and balloon out, death can result. If the brain's covering membranes or its bony protective case—the skull—are damaged, the brain itself can be damaged past healing. A headache can herald all these conditions and others.

But the lack of a headache does not mean those conditions do not exist; in other words, you cannot depend upon a headache to warn you that such dangerous conditions are present. Hypertension—high blood pressure—is called the "silent killer" because it rarely causes headaches or other warning symptoms.

Your systolic blood pressure (the top number of blood pressure readings) has to top 180 or so, for instance, before it precipitates a headache, and it may not even then. Yet systolic pressures of less than 180 are high enough to pose a dangerous potential for stroke and other problems with blood vessels.

Joan's full medical workup revealed nothing remarkable. She enjoyed normal health when she wasn't stricken with migraine. Now we were ready to launch into a program of treatment to alleviate Joan's problem and, by extension, Mark's. In recording the process, we hope to show you how you can alleviate your headache pain.

Let us look first at the different kinds of headaches and what they are doing to Joan and Mark—and to you.

CHAPTER **2**

How Headaches Happen

Find out why headaches occur?" Joan looked skeptical. "Why do I want to know how they happen? All I want is some kind of medicine that will prevent them from happening again." She sat in my office looking a thousand percent better than she had a week ago. Gone were the bathrobe and the hangdog expression. Her blonde hair bounced like a shampoo commercial. She wore a delicate pink sweater that flattered her natural coloring, and her eyes sparkled.

The migraine had passed, as migraines always do. Joan was bright, alert, and cheerful. Mark even seemed more chipper than before, simply because his wife was feeling good.

I answered her question with an illustration. "Let's say you're driving around town doing errands, and your car begins to cough and sputter. You just manage to get it off the road before the engine quits. Now, two people stop to help you. The first one says, 'I know what's wrong. It's your whatzit. I'll call a tow truck and they can tow you to my shop and I'll replace your whatzit for three hundred dollars.' The second one says, 'It's not the whatzit, it's the whoozit. I'll connect these two little wires directly, instead of through the whoozit, and you can be on your way.' "

She smiled. "I think I met those two. I'll just call Mark."

"Mark isn't available."

"Oh. Well . . ."

I pressed on. "If you know what the whoozit does, you'll know whether it's safe to avoid the whoozit by rewiring."

"I gotcha!" She brightened. "And if I know what the whatzit does, I'll probably know whether it's the whatzit causing the problem. Or at least I'll know it can't be the whatzit."

"Exactly."

Similarly, the more you know about how the head functions physiologically, the better you can understand what you and your doctor are trying to do for headache management. This is not to say doctors know all about it. We are in the dark in many ways as to what really goes on during a headache. Historically, we have plenty of company in our uncertainty.

The Ghosts of Headaches Past

Five thousand years ago, people from the cradle of Western European civilization, Mesopotamia, were writing chants and poems about migraines. They assigned the cause to an evil spirit, Tiu. And why not? Who else but an evil spirit would strike so low a blow?

Archaeologists exploring the Inca civilization of South America found human skulls with holes cut in them, a treatment technique called *trepanning* or *trephining*. New bone had grown around the holes, indicating that the patients not only survived their brain surgery but lived for years thereafter. Possibly to cure migraines, someone apparently hit upon the idea of providing an exit route for malevolent spirits. Trepanning was also practiced in Mesopotamia.

"No. Huh-uh. Not me." Mark winced at the thought of cutting holes in his head.

"I can understand their desperation. When the migraine really begins to bear down," Joan mused, "I believe I just might be ready to try drilling holes."

Alfred Nobel and Alexander Graham Bell, Sigmund Freud and Woodrow Wilson, George Bernard Shaw and Julius Caesar, John Calvin and Kareem Abdul-Jabbar all, like Joan, suffered excruciating, recurring migraines. No culture, no period of history, has ever been free of the malady. It is not a uniquely modern problem.

But migraine is not the only debilitating headache. The man (or much less frequently, woman) suffering cluster headaches will tell you nothing hurts worse. He may be right. Then there are tension headaches, the most common sort, which vary widely in severity from "dull throb" to "bison stampede." We have identified scores of other kinds that occur less frequently. The one thing they share in common is misery.

Your head may or may not be the origin of the headache. It certainly is the location of it. Yet it's not your brain that's hurting. Without getting into specialized terms like *pia mater* and *dura mater*, let's look at some basic anatomy.

The Brain and Nervous System

Picture Mark on a winter morning in Cleveland. To drive to work he must free his car from the clutches of last night's snowfall and low temperature. He stomps out through two inches of new snow, digs the windshield scraper out from under the seat, and mutters little phrases like, "Bah, humbug," and "In Miami, it's seventy-seven degrees."

Almost instantly, Mark's fingers get so cold they hurt. While he struggles in valiant hand-to-hand combat with Mother Nature, he reviews the workday before him and makes a mental note to stop by the Magic Money Machine at the bank and withdraw forty dollars so that he has cash for lunch.

His nose starts to run. By the time he's inside the car urging the reluctant motor to life, his feet are very, very cold. Suddenly he becomes aware that that one cup of coffee he's had so far isn't nearly enough to get him through the morning. His fingers are so stiff that he has trouble handling his handkerchief to blow his nose. As Mark scrapes ice and grinds the car's starter, a lot is going on inside of him, most of which he is blissfully unaware.

Inside Mark

If Mark's skull were solid it would be almost too heavy to lift. Fortunately, it's hollow. The biggest hollow space is the main cavity where the brain resides. You've seen a drawing of a cross section of the human head in high school biology, back when you didn't care all that much. You know the brain is in there.

Directly behind your forehead and around your

eyes and up behind your nose are other smaller cavities, the sinuses. These spaces allow the skull to protect your brain the way it's supposed to do without weighing a lot. The sinuses are lined with smooth tissue that keeps itself moist (sometimes too moist, it would seem, as Mark can attest when he experiences his sinuses draining).

Numerous little holes and passages allow specific, specialized nerves to connect between the brain and your sense organs. These cranial (*cranium* means *skull*) nerves occur in a particular order which medical students must memorize as one of their first exercises in anatomy. The olfactory nerve connects to the nose and receives smells, the auditory nerve connects to the ear and receives sounds, the optic nerve connects to the eye, and so on. One of these nerves, which serves the face, is the trigeminal. It will play a special part in certain headaches.

The skull perches on top of the backbone, or spinal column. The backbone is actually a lot of bones, called *vertebrae*, stacked upon each other and tied together with extremely strong, tough fibers like strings of thick plastic. Each vertebra has a hole down through it. The holes line up vertically so that the thick spinal cord can run from the brain, through a big hole in the skull, and down the inside of the stacked vertebrae of the spinal column. Along the whole length of this complex, nerves run out from the spinal cord, like branches on a tree, to all the many parts of the body they serve.

Cord is a somewhat misleading word, for the brain, nerves, and spinal cord are neither tough nor strong. In fact, they're not much stronger than set gelatin.

However, picture wrapping a block of gelatin very snugly in plastic wrap. Thus enclosed, the gelatin actually becomes fairly durable. It keeps its shape, even when pressed upon, and doesn't sag much. The nerves, brain, and spinal cord are similarly wrapped in very thin, very tough membranes: *dura mater*, *arachnoid*, and *pia mater*, collectively called *meninges*. These membranes provide strength and help the nerves, brain, and cord keep their shape, and protect against injury.

The brain and spinal cord are hollow. A colorless fluid, the cerebrospinal fluid, circulates freely in the hollow space. Fluid also circulates between the layers of very thin membranes covering the brain itself.

Should your doctor recommend a lumbar puncture to test the cerebrospinal fluid for some abnormality, he is talking about tapping into the hollow space of the spinal cord with a needle to extract some of the freely circulating fluid. Because the fluid washes up through the brain, its chemical analysis can tell a doctor much about what's going on inside—particularly if there is some sort of infection present.

The brain with its emergent nerves and the spinal cord together comprise the central nervous system. But the nervous system cannot function in haughty aloofness. It requires an amazing and intricate support system.

The Supporting Players

"To keep your feet warm in cold weather, put on a hat," Mark's mom used to tell him. Now that he's old enough to ignore her, he disregards her advice. He should pay attention to it.

Cranial Nerves and What They Do

These nerves connect the brain to the outside world. Sensory nerves pick up information coming from the outside, and motor nerves direct activities of the organs to which they connect.

1. **PREOPTIC:**
   A small nerve, also called Terminal, at the very front; serves the front of the head.

2. **OLFACTORY:**
   A bundle of about twenty sensory nerves conveying smells and delicate aromas that the nose detects.

3. **OPTIC:**
   The sensory nerve exclusively devoted to your sense of sight. All visual information comes in through here.

4. **OCULOMOTOR:**
   The motor nerve directing eye movements.

5. **TROCHLEAR:**
   This smallest of the cranial nerves directs movement of the eye downward and outward.

6. **TRIGEMINAL:**
   The largest of the cranial nerves, this complex network sends feelings from your head and face to the brain. One branch, serving the jaw with both motor and sensory functions, also directs chewing. When an infection or irritation hits this nerve, you feel it!

7. **ABDUCENS:**
   This motor nerve serves muscles controlling the eyes.

8. FACIAL:

Facial expressions are directed by this complex motor nerve. It serves the scalp and sides of the neck as well. It also acts as a sensory nerve bringing in taste messages.

9. AUDITORY:

Connecting the cochlea and vestibule of your ear, it sends both hearing and balance messages to the brain.

10. GLOSSOPHARYNGEAL:

Glosso- is Tongue and *Pharynx/pharyngeal* refers to the upper throat parts, which tells you where this one goes. It delivers feeling and taste messages as well as performing motor functions.

11. VAGUS:

Some call it the Pneumogastric nerve, referring to the lungs (pneuma) and stomach (gastric). It coordinates the brain with the heart and lungs. It extends branches all through the neck, down to the lungs, and to the heart and stomach.

12. ACCESSORY:

. . . Accessory to the Vagus, specifically, it also connects with the spinal nerves below the brain.

13. HYPOGLOSSAL:

This nerve serves the deepest part of the tongue and hyoid area (where gills would open, if we had gills).

Below the Hypoglossal, the Spinal Nerves begin, leaving the spinal cord through openings in the neck and trunk vertebrae.

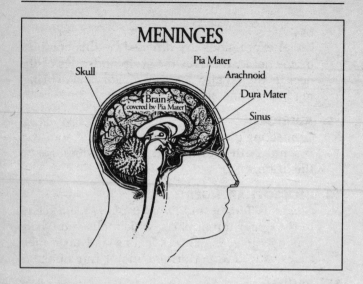

MENINGES

Pia Mater

Skull

Arachnoid

Dura Mater

Brain
covered by Pia Mater

Sinus

His brain is functioning fully as he scrapes and brushes snow. His hands are doing one thing as his brain works full-tilt on something else altogether—the workday and lunch. He plans what he's going to do with his day. He remembers he's low on pocket money. His brain will remind him as he passes the bank to pull in and hit up the automated teller. In other words, cold is not affecting his mental capacities. But it is affecting his peripheral circulation. As it happens, he is not wearing a hat today, and his hands and feet are indeed cold. Mark would be much more comfortable in a snug cap. His mom's axiom is not so farfetched; its principle works this way:

Because the nervous system is alive in every sense of the word, it needs a way to receive oxygen and get rid of wastes. The blood serves that function. So the brain with its extensive network of nerves receives a rich and constant supply of blood from an equally extensive network of blood vessels, arteries (bringing oxygen-rich blood), and veins (hauling away waste-laden blood). The blood, because it circulates deeply, rises to core body temperature inside, and then carries that body heat around with it. If your hands or feet get really cold, as Mark's do when he is scraping the frost off his windshield, the tiny blood vessels in them simply tighten up. Less blood flows through the extremities, and therefore less blood volume is cooled by the cold flesh. The process conserves body heat.

But your brain, which needs that constant supply of oxygen, cannot operate with less blood, no matter how cold it gets. So the major blood vessels in your head constrict very little. As the blood circulates merrily up there, its proximity to the cold outside cools it off, and you lose body heat. Hence the need for a hat to keep your blood—and thereby your feet and other parts—cozy and warm.

This relative inability to constrict can exacerbate other problems. If you suffer a severe accident and major blood vessels in your head are ripped or punctured, they tend to bleed long and profusely because they cannot close down as well as the veins and arteries of your arm or leg. This problem is true for internal bleeding as well as bleeding you can see.

And what about swelling? Really bang your shin and you can show off the bruise (actually internal bleeding) and the swollen bump. Should you bang your head, you'll have a bump to show for it, and perhaps a bruise. But if the internal bleeding—bruising—and enlarged bump occur inside the skull, there is nowhere for the blood and swelling to go, no space for expansion. The swelling puts pressure on the brain itself, and that pressure can damage or destroy vital brain cells.

Blood vessels themselves are little more than leaky garden hoses. They have tiny holes which widen or constrict through the efforts of thin little sheets of muscle that surround them. Those muscles are cued by tiny nerves. The cold triggered the vessels in Mark's fingers to close down so much that he's temporarily lost both feeling and dexterity. Only when his hands warm again will they regain their normal function.

Mark did not consciously decide to close down his peripheral circulation. This was done by a special set of nerves, the *autonomic system*. As the term implies, it functions pretty much automatically, separate from conscious thought. The autonomic nerves march to a different drummer—not conscious thoughts but rather perceived problems and physical conditions.

You are beginning to see, I trust, the marvelous complexity of your body and of all the intricate actions and reactions that occur when you do something as simple as scrape a windshield. When anything goes wrong to alter normal reactions or even to speed them up, a headache sometimes results.

A number of factors are going to affect Mark today. At work, he will face an unanticipated load of emergency jobs that will destroy his carefully laid plans. He will have to put up with an annoying coworker, an obtuse boss who doesn't understand him, and a long commute. His muscles normally tighten up when anxiety, anger, and frustration rise; everyone's do. His will do so today. In addition, he'll have Chinese food at noon; he doesn't know his body reacts adversely to the monosodium glutamate in his stir-fry.

If Mark tries to compensate for the tension by exercising strenuously, he will do himself no favors if he's one of those people for whom sudden strenuous exercise triggers headaches. Thanks to the effect of all these stresses and frustrations pulling his intricately tuned body a little out of tune, Mark is ripe for a dandy of a brain-buster.

Where the Pain Comes From

During Mark's afternoon coffee break, the dull throb started. Now, at four P.M., he thinks his brain is exploding. The heaviness at the back of his head has grown into thick pain in back and front.

Actually, his brain doesn't feel a thing. The brain itself has no nerves that identify or transmit pain. The brain cannot sense anything by itself; it reads only what incoming sensory nerves tell it. Pain sensors outside the brain are telling Mark about his headache.

The damp Ohio cold this morning did not precipitate his headache, though he may suspect it did. Tense muscles, both the muscles of his neck, head, and shoulders and the muscles controlling his blood vessels, will contribute to the headache. We don't know the exact physiological cause of muscle tension headaches, but we certainly see the effect.

In certain headaches, the thin sheets of muscle around the blood vessels tighten and then let go, expanding outward. Suddenly, blood that was being compressed has lots of room to move in the larger vessels. The rapid change in blood pressure, we suspect, contributes to the headache, though we're not certain just how.

Infections in the thin saran-like membranes that wrap the brain and spinal cord can cause headaches. So can spontaneous bleeding—that is, bleeding from an internal blood vessel rupture rather than from an externally caused wound. And of course, trauma from without can produce a headache, as anyone who has suffered an accident knows.

The support systems in Mark's head, then, have turned against him. His muscles and blood supply, thrown off kilter, are generating an ache in his head, even though the large majority of his head is occupied by the unfeeling brain. And, of course, it works that way for you, too.

What's Happening, Man?

Joan listened patiently to an explanation of the physiological processes associated with her head and wrinkled her nose. "That's all very good, but now what?"

Knowing what's happening is helpful in several very important ways. The more you understand the physiology of what is going on inside you, the better you can help your doctor find an answer to your headaches. You enter into the process not as a passive subject but as an informed partner. When he asks what a particular course of treatment is doing for you, you can help with knowledgeable answers. When he describes what he wants to do, you can pick up on his explanation.

22 · · · · · · · · · · · · · ·

With this knowledge, you can better envision what a particular medicine is supposed to be doing for you. When your doctor describes a drug as a *vasoconstrictor*, you understand that it is supposed to close down the blood vessels, or perhaps simply keep them from dilating, and you now know that's done by controlling those tiny muscles on the vessel walls. A *vasodilator* performs the opposite effect. If you're not sure what a medicine does, ask!

If you are not under a doctor's care, understanding these physiological processes is even more important. As this book discusses each kind of headache, it will offer charts and tables to help you pinpoint what is affecting you. You could simply memorize: " 'Tension headache; often starts at the back of the head.' Okay. I've got that down." Or you could understand: "I see. It figures that a tension headache might often start at the back; that's where the tightening, tensing muscles of the neck and shoulders are contracting." If it makes sense, you'll remember it a whole lot longer.

Most important, knowing what's happening puts you on what might be called an intelligent alert for danger signs. As we examine the various kinds of headaches, their causes, and their management, we'll discuss important danger signals in detail. We'll then summarize them in the end.

Pain, including headache pain, is actually very useful. ("Oh, sure," groans Joan.) It warns you that something needs adjustment or correction. Those extremely rare persons with little or no pain sensation may elicit envy at first glance. ("They certainly do from me," says Joan wistfully.) But should something dangerous or even lethal go wrong within their bodies, they have virtually no way of knowing about it.

Headache sufferers, then, are blessed. In dealing with their headaches, they will have to deal with the problem or disease that is causing it, and in the end they will be much healthier for the experience. This includes improved health of body, of mind, and of spirit.

Joan's first step was to undergo the medical workup. The second step will be to alleviate her pain on a temporary basis, usually with appropriate medicines. Like other typical headache sufferers, Joan will not be able to deal effectively with root causes if she is distracted by pain.

The third step, then, will be to uncover the root causes in order to either end, or at least greatly curtail, headache recurrences. This step is the most difficult and ultimately the most rewarding. It will require some detective work, perhaps some experimentation, and a lot of introspection. It almost certainly will mean altering her lifestyle to some degree.

Joan frowns. "You're saying I'm going to have to give something up, right? Something I probably like a lot, like chocolate."

Every person is different. Therefore, every life-style alteration will be tailored to fit that person. That's where the detection comes in. Joan has a unique problem; she must uncover the solution that works for her.

Quite possibly, a headache sufferer cannot do that detection well without a doctor's help. Consider also that there are situations and conditions that require medical intervention immediately. Let's pause in the consideration of Joan's misery and look at what a doctor asks his patient. Let's also look at what danger signs physicians particularly look for.

(Incidentally, after you've read the book, come back to this next chapter and skim through it again. It will mean much more the second time through, after you have a wider understanding of the different kinds of headaches and what causes them to happen.)

CHAPTER 3

What the Doctor Will Look For

My dear," she cooed, "of course you're depressed!" This older lady had read all the books. She was confident she knew the psychological signs when she saw them. She understood getting in touch with yourself and all the latest. She herself needed no further improvement, but she recognized the various signs in all her neighbors and knew just what advice to give them. As her blue hair glowed in the sunlight, Eve hung over the back fence and dispensed volumes of unrequested advice to her neighbor, Jeanne.

Jeanne listened to Eve. She had to admit that Eve knew all the terminology. And Eve had described Jeanne's situation to a tee. Jeanne felt slack. She lacked energy. She suffered frequent tension headaches. She felt no pleasure in living and no enthusiasm for activities that used to give her great joy. Jeanne was approaching middle age, a fact which didn't please her in the slightest; and since she'd been a housewife for so many years, she was probably unemployable now.

Eve burbled on. "A severe depression is to be expected, Jeanne. After all, your youngest just left home for college. Your husband changed jobs recently; the new hours are a drain after you were so used to his old routine. All sorts of factors."

"I suppose so." Jeanne still felt dubious. "All my friends say the same thing. Empty nest and all that. But I'm glad the kids are all finally on their own. I can't imagine being depressed by an empty nest. I mean—"

"Well, you just trust your friends, dear. We know best. We've all been through it. I'll give you that book on depression and you read it, and you'll be fine again."

Jeanne almost took Eve's advice. The "almost" saved her life. Jeanne's severe depression was caused by an operable tumor.

How did Jeanne know to go to the doctor? How did the doctor know to look for something beyond depression or a simple tension headache? The answer is complex. Let's examine it by looking at what the doctor will want to know when you visit.

The Doctor's First Questions

When Jeanne rather tentatively sat down with her doctor, she wasn't sure this visit was necessary. Everyone gets headaches. She got headaches. Her headaches had become much more frequent recently, but as Eve and others assured her, that was to be expected. Her life had just changed drastically.

Her doctor's evaluation was focused on three areas of inquiry: a personal history, a physical examination, and any laboratory tests the history and examination suggested.

When you see a physician to discuss the management

of your headache, the doctor's evaluation can only be as good and as accurate as the information you provide. I suggest that you write down the answers to these questions in advance and have them in hand when you go in. Jeanne did so, and it helped immensely.

"I'd forget my head if it wasn't attached," she griped. "When I go in and actually sit down, I don't remember half of what I ought to tell the doctor. By writing down things as I think of them over a period of a couple of days, I don't forget them in the doctor's office."

1. Your age, job, marital status, current stressful happenings in your life, etc.

2. How your headache first starts to come on

3. Exactly where in your head you feel your headache pain

4. Is there other pain as well—in your neck, for instance?

5. How long have you been suffering from these headaches? Days? months? years?

6. How frequently do they occur?

7. Has there been a change in the frequency of your headaches? Describe.

8. About how long does each episode last?

9. Is there a pattern to their occurrence? (For example, do they happen in clusters? Do they always occur around the same time of month? on weekends? after sex or other strenuous exercise? when you're especially tired?)

10. Do the episodes occur about the same time of day? Are they more pronounced as the day progresses, or do you wake up with them in the morning and they subsequently abate? Do they come on slowly or subside slowly?

11. Describe the nature of the pain. Is it throbbing? pressing? stabbing? dull? hideous? Does the pain change, or stay the same?

12. Do certain actions aggravate the pain? Sneezing? coughing? turning your head quickly? bending over? standing up?

13. What other symptoms occur at the same time or just before onset? Flashing lights or other aural phenomena? watery eyes? nausea? diarrhea? excessive irritability?

14. How do you fight them? Do you use over-the-counter analgesics? Cold packs? Rest? Were these methods effective?

15. What did you try in the past that did not work?

16. What other medications are you on now? (This includes birth control pills as well as prescription medicines.) Don't forget to list "special diets" or over-the-counter medicines.

17. Have you been diagnosed as having other ailments? What are they? Are they under control?

18. Is anything going on in your life that disturbs you? (It could be physical or emotional or outside yourself.)

19. Are you being seen by any other doctor?

20. Who else in your family (we're particularly concerned with blood relatives) suffers headaches? What are their headaches like?

I might mention a few points of explanation about some of these questions. Your age is important. For example, temporal (an irritation of the arteries in the temple area) arteritis is fairly common among older people, rare among the young. Trigeminal neuralgia (stabbing facial pain) rarely occurs before age thirty-five. So when a headache is not age appropriate, we look more closely.

The location of the pain also tells a great deal. It tells the doctor approximately what nerves, sinuses, and other anatomical structures are involved. With information about the location and the kind of pain, your doctor can sort out how many different kinds of headaches you suffer from. Migraineurs get tension headaches like everyone else, and people suffering tensions headaches may be subject to other kinds as well. People experiencing cluster headaches usually are refractory between episodes—that is, they are headache free until and unless the clusters strike. All this information is diagnostic.

We have found that the longer you've been burdened with these miseries (see question 5), the better the chance that they are benign. Long-time chronic headaches usually do not indicate dangerous conditions. A noticeable change in frequency, particularly an abrupt change in frequency, however, is a big red flag. This change is what brought Jeanne in to her doctor.

Answers to questions 9 and 10, describing the patterns of occurrence, help the doctor a great deal. Give them careful thought.

If you mention a cough in question 12, that too is a red flag. Sneezing, coughing, bending, or straining that precipitates a headache or intensifies a headache suggests brain problems. The cough headache lasts a few minutes or less. However, 10 percent of persons who experience brief cough headaches may show intracranial lesions or certain other malformations.

In question 13, a *prodrome*—that is, a series of odd phenomena preceding a headache—is a finger pointing to migraine. Cluster headaches may cause the eye on the affected side to water and puff up. These clues are all what we call giveaways.

Different kinds of headaches respond to different kinds of treatment (see question 14). If a certain treatment works when others do not, that is a clue to the kind of headache you're dealing with.

Medications mentioned in question 16 are extremely important for your doctor to know about. Some medicines may work against the medicine your doctor plans to prescribe. He should know about any you take. Some, such as birth control pills, may contribute to your headache. Any medicines you take, including over-the-counter remedies, alter your body chemistry. Your doctor must know about that.

Asking about other doctors in question 19 is not out of jealousy or rivalry. We all have to work together. And that means we all have to know who on the team is doing what.

Picture harnessing a team of Clydesdales to a heavily loaded wagon. One horse alone weighs nearly a ton. If these horses work together as a team, they can pull an amazingly large load. Now picture each of them either not knowing what the others are doing or not caring. They pull in different directions. Some stop. Some eat grass. Some cast eyes upon the others with amorous intent. Your loaded wagon is not going to go very far very well. You and your doctor or doctors constitute a team, just like a team of horses. The better the teamwork, the better the results.

We ask question 20 because predisposition to certain headaches runs along family lines in two ways. It could be a genetic predisposition, as migraine may be. Even though we have no clear handle on why migraine occurs, it seems to run strongly along family blood lines. Also, a person's earliest training and subliminal thinking is shaped by family attitudes and values. For instance, many people learn subconsciously that the way to garner attention or win a debate is to have a headache. That's what the older family members did; therefore that must be the way. None of this thought process is conscious. It's programmed in. But it still causes a headache. Much depends upon family history and predisposition.

The Physical Examination

When Jeanne's doctor tested her knee reflexes, she started getting a little perturbed. Jeanne sniffed. "Honestly. There she was, examining every other part of my body except my head. I was thinking to myself, 'Who cares if my leg flies up in the air?' I was there for frequent headaches.

"I understand now. As my doctor explained it, all

the other body parts and functions connect into the brain. By seeing which parts function well and which do not, you get some idea of what's happening in the brain. Still, I thought at first that she was just being overly thorough."

Besides looking at whether reflexes and coordination indicate some sort of brain problem, we check for symmetry in reflexes and nerve function. Your hands should squeeze with equal strength. Your two knees should show equal reactions to stimuli.

Physicians are very good at recognizing a simple indicator: "Does the patient *look* sick?" As subjective as that sounds and as hard to describe or define as it may be, it tells us whether the patient's blood flow to various organs is adequate and gives us other important clues.

As your doctor works through your own medical examination, he or she may find something that requires closer scrutiny. We are blessed with a variety of diagnostic tests and machines to help us see beyond the formerly impenetrable barrier of the skull and into the deepest inner workings of your body.

Tests

Various X rays and brain scanning techniques help us spot abnormalities. Electroencephalograms and electrocardiograms (EEGs and EKGs) tell us whether normal patterns of nerve activity have been altered. They are extremely useful.

Thorough laboratory blood testing provides us with a wealth of useful information. Now and then we'll do a spinal tap to test the fluid circulating inside your central nervous system. No test is used by itself. Each has its shortcomings. But taken all together, the tests and probes can give us a helpful picture of unusual happenings and physical problems.

In Jeanne's case, a CAT scan (Computer-Assisted Tomography, a type of X ray) identified a tumor the size of an egg. Other tests confirmed it. Fortunately, it was placed so that the neurosurgeon could remove it cleanly.

Reading Your Body

Jeanne's situation provides a cautionary tale, and it concerns that old saw "Everybody knows." Everybody knew that Jeanne's problem was a simple case of the blues because her kids were out on their own. Everybody knew that if it really were a brain tumor, she'd have a pounding headache in the place where the tumor lay. Everybody knew a tumor causes partial paralysis, or extreme mood swings, or insanity, or some other drastic indication—not mild depression.

Jeanne listened not to "everybody knows" but to her body. And she won the game.

In fact, most of what everybody knows is not true. The vast majority of headache complaints are nothing more than that—simple headaches. On the other hand, headaches accompany only one-third of all tumors and similar problems. Most remain "silent."

Even when a headache is a symptom of a tumor or other brain problem, the problem is often not severe. Remember that the brain itself feels nothing, so the location of the pain is not a solid clue as to the location of a tumor. And don't count on mood swings and other emotional or physical problems to tell you there's trouble. Certainly, they sometimes show up, and when they do you must immediately pay attention to them. But a lot of nasty things can go on inside you with no outward sign. And a lot of headaches can make your day miserable although there is no serious underlying problem.

Danger Signals

Jeanne's clue, a marked increase in frequency of tensionlike headaches, was vague at best. Not really black and white. Most clues are like that and they're easily overlooked. Your best bet by far for picking up on real dangers early is simply to be able to read your body well.

Jeanne commented, "I've learned that if you notice a body part, something's wrong." She's right.

Think how, from day to day, you go about your activities. You don't consciously think that you are moving your legs as you walk across the room or that your feet are now walking on linoleum whereas before they were on carpeting. Your hand reaches for a can in the cupboard, your fingers close around it, and you don't even think about it. You're thinking about whether to put just this one can of tomato paste in this batch of lasagna sauce or to open two cans.

But if your knuckles hurt as you close your hand around the can or if your feet ache as you walk across the carpet, you are aware that something is wrong. You may have arthritis that limits your hand function or feet that are tired from your being on them all day. The condition could be benign or serious, but you notice.

Be that aware in regard to headaches as well. Most

are benign. But we can't safely assume that they are harmless 100 percent of the time.

We consider these specific signs to be an indication that a closer look is necessary and should be done quickly:

A severe headache that strikes suddenly. The vast majority of sudden-onset headaches are harmless. The doctor should look for the rare case in which the sudden headache indicates bleeding inside the skull. We refer to blood seepage from certain types of blood clots as minibleeds. Minibleeds are often precursors to massive bleeds occurring not long after. If your doctor can catch the minibleed, therefore, the patient enjoys excellent chances for recovery. Fortunately, minibleeds usually cause severe headaches; you just know something bad is going on.

Heavy bleeding beneath one of the brain's protective membranes, called a subarachnoid hemorrhage, has nowhere to go. The freed blood mixes with cerebrospinal fluid and exerts fluid pressure on adjacent brain cells, causing severe damage quickly. A CAT scan for lesions is your best chance of spotting problems of this sort and should be done quickly.

Any headache that causes what we call neurological deficit—a problem of the brain or nerves not functioning well. Your vision blurs or is reduced in some way; you feel tingling or paralysis in some body area; you have trouble speaking clearly or remembering words; the headache causes you confusion or a decreased level of consciousness; your hearing dulls—these are common neurological deficits but not a complete list.

Any headache that is intensified if you bend over, sneeze, cough, or turn your head quickly.

Headaches that come to older persons who were relatively headache free previously. They may not be simply "the price of getting older."

Convulsions. All convulsions are red flags. But any convulsions following a blow on the head must be investigated instantly. Don't wait a minute on this one.

Headache with fever. Here's another sign you evaluate immediately, especially in children. Fever is an indication of infection—some sort of bacterial microbe has invaded, and the body responds by warming up several degrees. Meningitis and any of a number of infectious agents attacking the central nervous system can cause coma, death, or permanent debilitation and can cause them quickly. Our best indication of meningitis is sudden onset of fever, neck pain, and headache. Often, nausea appears as well. A telltale clue is stiffness or pain at the back of the neck. In extreme cases, the sufferer lies arched backward in a "C" position.

Frequently recurring headaches in children.

An abrupt change in the pattern or location of "common" headaches. Medically evaluate any such changes. Check out changes in frequency, as Jeanne did.

Heavy malaise. Some malaise is natural. Of course you feel rotten, even with a so-called simple tension headache. Here I'm talking about extreme loss of alertness. Mental confusion should not be considered a symptom of a normal headache either.

Any headache that wakes you up at night.

Before you panic, keep in mind that danger signals are never a guarantee that something terrible is going wrong. They are clues to a possible problem and nothing more. For example, like Jeanne, Gwen experienced a sudden change in the number and the intensity of the migraines she had been suffering for half her life. Like Jeanne, she saw a doctor about it. Let me emphasize that both women acted correctly. In Gwen's case, that danger signal pointed to no problem whatever. Migraines occasionally do shift frequency. Hers did, harmlessly. But she was very wise to get evaluated.

The Doctor's List

Jeanne snorted in disbelief. "Wait. You're saying that doctors have a list of all the kinds of headaches? But I thought different people have different levels of pain response. What is terrible pain for me might be mild for someone else. How can you make an objective list?"

"Grab your forearm with your other hand and dig in your fingernails firmly," Jeanne's doctor, Meg Rosen, began. "Feel it? Call that level one pain. Very mild. Now think back on the most excruciating pain you ever felt. Call that a ten. Do you see how we do it?"

"I see. My perception might be different from someone else's, but everyone's scale is the same."

"Exactly. But with a caveat." Dr. Rosen smiled. "Think of a little child who's about to get a shot. The child thinks it's going to hurt. He's afraid it will hurt. Therefore it's going to hurt. My nurse can get a howl of pain from some little kids before the needle is anywhere close to them. So there's a strong psychological component that you have to factor in to pain analysis.

"Not only do we have a list that classifies all the kinds of headaches, we give them numbers. Here. I'll show you." She brought out a small handbook by the Headache Classification Committee of the International Headache Society.

Jeanne laughed. "This is worse than the Dewey Decimal System I had to learn in school!"

"But that's exactly the idea." Dr. Rosen opened the book at random to a page. Here was item 1.3, Ophthalmoplegic migraine. Under that, it offered:

A. At least two attacks fulfilling B.

B. Headache overlapping with paresis of one or more of cranial nerves III, IV, and VI.

C. Parasellar lesion ruled out by appropriate investigations.

This headache classification is not just academic. Insurance companies and others in addition to doctors, use it at least in part. For example, some insurance companies cover TIA's—transient ischemic attacks, item 6.1.1—and others do not.

The list begins with migraine, item 1., for a reason. Migraines cost billions yearly in lost work time, and that dollar figure is only the measurable impact. Worse still are the suffering and depression migraines generate.

Our friend Joan entered treatment with some skepticism, but she entered. The sheer misery of her migraines drove her to it. Let's therefore start out with an examination of Joan's problem: the vicious, intense, clamoring, debilitating headache called migraine.

I have included a simplified headache chart on the next pages so that you can get a quick overview of the many different types of headaches. We will talk about them individually in the following chapters.

Headaches Compared

	Migraine	Cluster	(CPH) Chronic Paroxysmal Hemicrania	Tension	Trauma (accident, etc.)	Trigeminal neuralgia
Nature of pain	Severe, enervating	Excruciating	Excruciating	Dull, pressing	Dull, pressing	Stabbing, sharp
Location	One side of head, temple behind eye	One side only	One side only	At back, or all around	General, not necessarily at injury site	Along temple side of head/face
Lasts for . . .	Few hours to few days	15–90 minutes per episode or cluster of episodes	1–2 minutes per episode or cluster of episodes	Few hours, few years	Days	Few seconds
Possible accompanying symptoms	May be preceded by aura; photophobia, sonophobia, nausea			Irritability	Dizziness, disequilibrium, blurred vision, loss of memory and concentration, unstable emotions	
Other notes	Prostrates sufferer	Sufferer paces, goes wild with pain				
Medications	Beta blocker prevents; Sumatripan, Ergotamine products, Antidepressants	Lithium Prednisone	Indomethacin	Non-prescription		

Headaches Compared

	Meningitis, other infection	Hematomis, hemorrhages	Temporal arteritis	Hangover, substance use	Sinus	Depression	Tumors
Nature of pain	Dull, pressing	Solid, growing, can change with position shift	Stabbing, sharp	Heavy, energy-draining	Tight, dull	Dull, pressing	Fluctuates
Location			Along temple, side of head/face	All Over!	Behind face: a "mask of pain"	At back, all around	Varies
Lasts for . . .		Varies	Varies	Hours	Usually hours	Varies	Varies
Possible accompanying symptoms	Stiff neck*	Worse when moving, stooping over*	Loss of vision*				Worse when moving, stooping over*
Other notes					Worst in A.M.	Wake up with it, it stays or worsens	
Medications			Tegretol	Non-prescription		Antidepressants	

*See Doctor immediately

CHAPTER 4

Migraine, Part I: What's Going On

Thomas Jefferson's migraine headaches sometimes lasted six weeks. He was luckier in a way than most migraineurs: he was able to work to some degree even while in the throes of misery. His headaches disappeared when he left the presidency.

Ulysses S. Grant, in the grip of a monstrous migraine, received the note of surrender from Lee. The Army of Northern Virginia was giving up. The bloody, interminable Civil War was ending. Grant's headache disappeared instantly.

Does this mean that it's all in your head? If Joan simply got rid of whatever stress point was plaguing her, would she suffer no more? Oh, if only it were so simple! If only some thought-change or magic pill could turn off the intense pain. It doesn't work that way.

What does work nearly all the time (nothing in medicine bears an iron-clad guarantee) is a combination of drug therapy to control the pain, thought or life-style change to control the source of tension, and attention to the details of emotional and spiritual welfare. By bringing all the patient's needs and dimensions into play, physician and patient together effect the cure.

We therefore urge any migraine sufferer to seek medical help if the steps suggested in this book do not seem to be working.

If you have never experienced a migraine, you cannot begin to appreciate the signs (what others see in you) and symptoms (what you feel yourself) Joan had to deal with. The symptoms vary from sufferer to sufferer, but there are some common features.

The Identifying Signs and Symptoms

Not even the migraineurs themselves may realize that symptoms begin up to two days before the headache itself strikes. The symptoms are little things, easily overlooked or disregarded.

You may feel depressed, as if nothing on earth is going your way, and nervous and irritable. Or instead you might feel especially great, on top of the world. You might be weary, totally pooped, or extremely energetic. You might get especially hungry or lose your appetite. In other words, you're living at extremes somehow. You're thirsty and you yawn a lot. Often, the people close to you notice these signs more than you do. You may not realize you feel all that unusual.

And then the axe falls, and the "classic" symptoms begin:

Pain

The throbbing, pulsating, severe pain may seem totally unbearable. It usually builds over minutes or hours and lasts less than 24 hours, although certain rare kinds can last three days or longer. It often occurs on one side of the head only, for example, over or around the right eye. The pain may shift to the other side during the course of the headache.

Walking up or down stairs often aggravates the pain, as may any other sudden movement or strenuous activity.

Occurrence

The migraineur may experience no symptoms at all for days or even years until the next occurrence. Women may find migraines associated closely with menstrual rhythms, the headaches occurring either before or during monthly periods. Joan did not suffer a migraine with every menstrual cycle. Some months were free of problems, other months brought intense headaches. Now and then a migraine would pounce on her unrelated to her cycle. Even though her headaches were partially predictable, their unpredictability weighed heavily. When would the next one strike?

Women experience migraines three times more frequently than do men. However, boys are affected during childhood. The headaches usually strike persons in their twenties, and they tend to fade as the migraineurs enter their fifties.

Many clients report that their migraines do not occur during times of high stress but rather afterward, as they relax—or try to. Many migraines occur shortly after awakening.

Accompanying Signs and Symptoms

Migraineurs may suffer nausea and vomiting before or during the headache. They may be rendered completely nonfunctional, as Joan was. Weakness may occur in an arm or a leg or in both limbs on one side.

Classic migraine, as they used to call it, brings with it an aura—that is, precursor symptoms to announce the misery's arrival, such as the visual phenomenon of flashing lights or wavy lines. Incidentally, doctors no longer call it classic. It's simply either migraine with aura or migraine without. A dull heaviness or sense of foreboding may also precede a migraine.

Women find that birth control pills can sometimes increase the frequency of migraines or worsen the pain. Blood pressure medicines may affect migraines as well.

During an episode, migraineurs report that bright lights or loud noises can drive them wild. Sometimes these symptoms immediately precede the episode.

After Effects

As just mentioned above, weakness may occur during an episode and usually passes when the headache does. But very rarely one side of the body can become permanently weakened by recurring migraines over time. Blood vessel constriction occurs with migraines. As those vessels close down tighter, they can choke off the nourishment of whatever body parts the blood vessels serve. Those body parts, oxygen-starved and waste-overloaded, are injured over and over again. With enough repetition of the injury, they can eventually become permanently damaged, somewhat reducing the strength of the affected body parts forever.

Recent studies indicate that peripheral vision can be permanently impaired as well. In other words, when you focus your eyes directly ahead of you, you cannot see as well off to the side, on the edge of your visual range. Not all migraineurs by any means will suffer these effects. Some do.

Sometimes the medicines used to combat migraine can cause dangerous side effects. There are times when the pain, excruciating as it is, may be more tolerable than the painkillers used to control it. Since there are dozens of medicines available you and your doctor should search for the right treatment for your unique migraine.

What triggers these devastating signs and symptoms?

Suspected Causes

We doctors could sound a lot more authoritative as we discuss migraine if we knew better why it happens. We aren't even sure just how it happens. Medical researchers in the '30s and '40s realized that blood vessels in the head changed size—closing down and dilating—and gave migraine the term *vascular headache*, meaning that the blood vessels were involved. You'll find migraine referred to as vascular headache in most literature.

Within the last ten years, researchers have been able to study in greater detail what goes on in the brain. They found that as the migraine begins, blood flow at the back of the brain is reduced. This region of reduced blood flow slowly spreads, like the fingers of mysterious glop in some horror movie until, two to six hours later, it has spread to about two-thirds of the brain area.

"Aha!" cry the theorists, "this suggests that the vascular effect is secondary and the headache is actually neurogenic in nature." That's fancy talk for saying that the blood vessel phenomenon is not a cause but an effect; some sort of nerve action or "misfiring" is the cause of the blood vessel changes.

That's important. When you treat the blood vessels, you're merely treating the symptoms of the headache. But if you treat the neurons themselves—the nerves— you are treating the cause. You're digging out the headache by its roots, so to speak, instead of simply pruning it. Keep this in mind as we proceed, for when we talk about drugs and cures in chapter five, we'll be looking at them in light of the "root" causes.

Other factors are involved in causing migraines, such as family history and personality type.

Up to seventy percent of migraineurs report that ancestors and others in their extended family suffered migraines as well. Dad got them, Mom did, uncles or aunts . . . .

"That's me!" Joan exclaimed. "My mother suffered for years. She often said she prayed I'd never be afflicted the way she was." And a shadow fell across her face. She shrugged and smiled wanly.

If you are a migraine sufferer like Joan, you're desperately trying to put your finger on the cause. Joan suspected her menstrual cycle because her headaches so frequently followed that time frame. Perhaps she was right. But most headaches are triggered by more than a single cause. Finding one cause does not preclude others.

Sigmund Freud came from a Jewish tradition. He suffered weekend migraines, frequently on Sundays. He felt that the anti-Semitic bias of the people around him, coupled with his unkind thoughts about the Christian Sabbath, triggered his bouts of misery. So it seems even our attitudes, thoughts, and worries can contribute to migraines as well.

In our clinical treatment, we have found all manner of possible and probable triggers. If you are a migraineur, ask yourself: "Do my headaches seem to occur when . . .

- . . . I become fatigued or I overexercise?"
- . . . I smoke before exercising?"
- . . . I sleep unusually late or find my sleep habits drastically altered for some reason?"
- . . . my allergies kick up?"
- . . . air pressure changes, as when a really big low pressure system (stormy weather) moves into the area?"
- . . . I encounter some known pollutant?"
- . . . I eat certain foods or classes of foods within the previous ten days?"
- . . . I go on, or have begun, certain medications?"
- . . . I have just been subjected to bright light?" (Light at concerts, discos, or movies—even bright sunlight—can be a factor.)

More than half the time, the migraine sufferer exhibits certain personality traits and behaviors. Do many of these characteristics describe you?

- Driven, relentless, out to get things done
- Like things to be just so; focus on details
- Rigid in actions and thinking; do not adapt easily
- Tend to keep people at a distance

- Ready to postpone pleasure today in order to advance future prospects; live for tomorrow
- Strong-willed, know what you want
- Expect the best from yourself and strive to achieve it
- Expect the best from others, too
- Tend to worry a lot
- Strong and in control emotionally
- Prefer to keep a strong grip on people, situations, and things around you, as well as on yourself

People exhibiting these characteristics tend to suffer migraine far more frequently than do more laid-back, casual sorts. Migraineurs tend to pride themselves on overachievement and extremely tight personal control. Whatever it is, they can handle it!

Sure they can.

How about you or the person you love? Do you fit the pattern of persons who are susceptible? Do the signs and symptoms sound like yours? Keep in mind here that the true migraineur need not suffer migraines exclusively. The migraineur is just as susceptible to other types of headaches as anyone else. Therefore, a better question is: Do any of your headaches fit these signs and symptoms?

As you may suspect, the mind-set I just described is almost certainly a contributing factor in migraines. The sufferers feel an intense need to appear strong, when in truth, down deep they feel insecure. Burying feelings always causes stress. Something has to give, so it may well manifest itself as a headache.

Sufferers who strive to appear superhuman—in fact, who strive to *be* superhuman—must necessarily deny their limitations. "I don't have any major limitations!" cries the typical migraineur. Mark referred to Joan as a powerhouse. She played tennis with him, went water-skiing, and made their camping excursions highly enjoyable experiences. She kept a neat house, volunteered with neighborhood service groups, served actively at church. Mark was proud of her. Joan could do anything!

Except when the headaches struck.

Persons who respond positively to the questions above often have a sense of worth based almost solely upon what they do or accomplish. They are goal oriented. If they don't put out, they consider themselves of little value. To succeed is to be worthy. These people have a strong statistical tendency to be migraineurs.

As I deal with migraineurs in a clinical setting, I very frequently find unresolved issues lurking within. These issues involve emotions and personal relationships.

Ambivalent feelings of self-worth are a part of it. The migraineur strives mightily to succeed, to achieve, to complete, to build, to . . . you get the idea. Episodes of migraine headache do not necessarily correspond to specific times of excessive stress. That does not mean this undercurrent of concern and doubt about self-worth do not play a major part.

Emotions also play a major part. In the personality profile I sketched above, the person is usually adept at hiding true emotions from others. That means the person almost certainly is also hiding true feelings from himself or herself. Persons who are overly controlling include their emotions in the list of things to be controlled.

Think for a moment about some film, book, or play that you would consider deeply touching. When I ask this of clients I sometimes get responses such as:

- "Naw, I never go to those kinds of flicks."
- "I don't like romantic stories. I'm more for action stuff."
- "Sorry. I limit my reading to serious nonfiction."

The overly controlling person will usually avoid entertainment that tugs at the heartstrings. To let loose, to shed a tear, to allow a film or book to manipulate you is to lose control. The person who routinely hides true emotions is understandably afraid of warm feelings; they cause a breakdown of control which bares those threatening emotions.

Control issues do not only affect the controller. The person in intense need to control literally overpowers the people closest to him or her. The wife submits to a controlling husband; the child chafes under heavy restrictions inappropriate to that child's age. Intimate personal relationships suffer greatly in both controller and controllee.

The mechanism works like this: the person controlled is torn between obedience and defiance. When the control is perceived as being overwhelming or inappropriate the defiance burns even stronger. With successful defiance come feelings of guilt that must either be denied or paid for, if they are acknowledged at all. When obedience wins the inner tussle, the person controlled feels intensely angry for being manipulated, for suffering perceived injustice. Anger in essence equals defiance, for it's certainly not a cooperative, amiable feeling. Greater efforts at obedience are required to offset this greater defiance/anger. Guilt and anger extract equally heavy prices in emotional stress. Around and down the spiral goes.

And while all this is going on, the controllers sense or even see outright that they cannot control the situations and people who concern them. They stand every moment on the brink of losing their hold. That's powerfully stressful to the person with a major need to be in control.

By these various mechanisms, then, excessive or inappropriate attempts at control generate severe stresses not just in the controller but in the person being controlled. You cannot get off by glibly saying, "That can't be it with me. I'm not a controlling type." You are still affected, and mightily so.

The stresses associated with this control dynamic very easily can trigger migraine. Where such stresses are a usual part of the interpersonal dynamic of close relationships, the headaches resulting from them will eventually become chronic and habitual.

How About You?

As we dig for stress sources, I would ask you about the following issues. Take a while and think about them.

Are You Being Controlled?

First, explore whether you are being controlled by someone else to the point that such control generates resentment (we're talking about adult to adult here, of course, not adults shaping or disciplining children. A child over fifteen is adult or nearly so):

- Do persons close to you tell you what to do and expect it to be done? Examples might be a husband telling his wife to discipline or redirect the kids or a wife telling her husband how to live his life: "Benson borrowed the mower? Well, you just go right over to Benson and get it back."
- Do persons close to you expect you to dress or behave in specific ways? "I don't want you wearing that hat." "When we get there, don't you dare head for the refreshment table."
- Do they attempt to manipulate you through guilt or wheedling? "All right; be that way. If I have a heart attack, it's your fault!" "If you really loved me you would _____!"
- If you saw the behavior those persons exhibit on a soap opera or on stage—at a distance, as it were— would you consider the behavior manipulative or controlling?
- If you saw that behavior elsewhere, would you expect the person being controlled to be angry or harbor resentment?
- Do persons close to you strongly resemble the personality I asked about in the section above?

Are You Controlling Others?

Now let's explore whether you yourself might be the controller (again, this is adult to adult):

- Do you expect to be followed or obeyed by those close to you?

- Did you give a positive response to the last item in the "Do many of these characteristics describe you" exercise?
- How about the question of expecting the best of others? Do you want to make certain they deliver it?
- Are you confident you know what is best for those closest to you? Are you annoyed when they are slow to respond to your efforts to help them do what is best?
- Do adults close to you ever appear annoyed or angry when you suggest they think or act in some particular way?
- Do you become angry or annoyed if others fail to follow your lead or suggestions?

Positive answers to these questions should tip you off that you or someone in your close circle of friends and relatives have a control problem of some degree. That can be a very strong stress point.

Joan and Mark pondered stress points, both in my office and as homework between sessions. Joan shook her head. "No, Mark isn't controlling. In fact he's very supportive. And I try hard not to be manipulative or nagging."

Mark assented. 'Joan's mom is a real Napoleon. If she had an army she'd rule the world. I'm proud of Joan that she recognizes her own tendency to be bossy and resists it so well."

"Mark even praises me when I hold my tongue."

I asked, "Would suppressing the desire to control be a stress point?"

She thought about that a minute. "No, I don't think so because no one is trying to hide it or anything. I'm not burying it. I'm just insisting to myself, 'This time, Joan, you're not going to tell Mark what to do.' I know the tendency is there. I'm exercising the free choice not to bow to it."

And that was the response I wanted from her. At that time it didn't matter one way or the other whether resisting her tendency was a source of stress. Rather, I wanted her and Mark both to examine the dynamics of their marriage and of their own motivations and behavior. I wanted them to see themselves as others would see them and to uncover problem areas. At this time we did not try to deal with problem areas and stress points. We simply identified them.

I enlisted Mark's help as much as hers because Joan's migraines affect not just her but also Mark and everyone else around her. It is not inappropriate in your own situation to talk to everyone close to you. What do they see as stress points? What do they suspect as possible causes of your headache? Tell them why you are asking these questions and solicit their help. Then listen to what they have to say.

Control issues did not loom large in the lives of Joan and Mark. But other issues did. Joan, you recall, was the classic achiever. She loved to accomplish. The moment she met one goal, she headed for the next. So I asked her, "If all of a sudden you ceased your work at church and your special projects and hired a housekeeper to clean and cook in your home, what would happen?"

She didn't hesitate a bit. "I'd go nuts."

"Why?"

"Because if I don't have something to do, I'll go nuts."

I sat back and folded my hands. "Explore the point. Why is doing—accomplishing—so important?" I wanted her to dig in and examine her actions and motivations at depth.

So should you.

Joan learned through long introspection that her reason for being was to accomplish. She was certain God could not use a person who just sits there. Now I had no intention of encouraging her to sit; neither did I intend to encourage her to achieve. We were probing the reasons for her actions. And her reasons surprised even her. She was worth nothing, she was sure, if she didn't have something to show for each day. That turned the thumbscrews and applied the pressure as nothing else could.

"Unless I can point to continual major accomplishments, I am nothing" was her subconscious motto. Powerful motivation. Powerful stress.

Mark was not achievement oriented in the same way or to the same degree, but he felt a strong need to prove his masculinity. He constantly had to be doing "guy things." For example, he kept the yard manicured perfectly, hauled the garbage, handled the recycling, tuned his car, and changed its oil. He never did dishes or housework, but Joan didn't care. He provided her an excellent dishwasher and floor polisher, which made her housekeeping go quicker and easier.

When she got migraines, Mark ended up with chores he perceived as unmanly, not to mention unfamiliar. There was a major source of tension for his tension headaches. The pieces of their puzzle were beginning to fall together.

You have a puzzle too. Not only must you fit pieces

together, you must first find them. Use every means you can to get a firm grip (there's that word again) on your motivations, expectations, and inner dynamics.

The Road to Cure

A friend of ours took her van to the dealer's service shop and explained what seemed wrong. "It's been acting sluggish for a while now. But out on the freeway today," she told the mechanic, "it began to buck and cough. Really buck! And the power just dropped to nothing. I was going thirty miles an hour with eighteen-wheelers crawling up my tailpipe. I can't drive it home this way."

He mused a while. "Let's start with the easiest first and put something in the gas tank to dry it out. If there's water in your fuel, your van will do that. The bucking especially."

It didn't help.

"We can try the fuel filter or the carburetor," he suggested. "The fuel filter is eight dollars and the sealed carb is four hundred."

"Try the fuel filter!"

They did. It worked.

It might appear that the mechanic was firing into the dark until eventually he hit something, but that's not so. There were, you see, four or five unrelated reasons why our friend's van might behave as it did. In fact, it could have been two or more conditions acting simultaneously. So the mechanic tried solutions according to a logical pattern: attempt the easiest and most obvious first, then go on to least costly, and finally try the most costly. As it turned out, her fuel filter was half full of water. Had that not been the case, she probably would have gone on to discover a faulty carburetor.

Doctors approach headache management in much the same way. There are a variety of possible causes for migraine and no way to tell which is the culprit. We try the easiest and most obvious first. If that produces no clear improvement, it's on to the next.

Migraine Headaches Compared with Tension Headaches

	Migraine	Tension
Onset	Sometimes preceded by aura	Gradual, builds
Pain	Severe, relentless	Tight, dull, maybe throbbing
Location	One side of head (might switch sides)	At back, or all around
Other Symptoms	Nausea, photophobia, sonophobia	Malaise; the blahs
Length of Headache	Half day to several days	A few hours, or nearly constant
Body's Response	Prostrated	Listless, slow but not stopped
Medications	Sumatriptan Ergotamines Beta blockers (preventative)	Over-the-counter aids: Aspirin Ibuprofen Acetaminophen

The same principle applies to medications. We try the simplest first. If that doesn't do the trick, we adjust dosages or try another prescription. We approach the problem methodically.

You, like Joan and Mark, have examined possible causes at length. Now let's move forward into a solution in the next chapter. Like the mechanic, we may have to try more than one thing. But we'll succeed!

CHAPTER 5

Migraine, Part II: The Cure

Nolan Ryan was on the mound for the Rangers, and the Mariners were already three runs down. It was a beautiful day . . . not necessarily a beautiful day for Seattle's team, but a lovely day here in Texas. Two friends, Cal and Paul, had brought their sons to the ballpark.

Cal's son asked for a hot dog, so Cal volunteered to make the refreshment run. "What'll you have?" he asked Paul.

Paul's boy requested a hot dog. Paul shook his head. "No thanks."

Cal gaped. "Baseball and hot dogs, Paul. You can't get along without a hot dog at the ballpark any more than you can get along without a glove compartment in your car. My treat."

"Wish I could, but hot dogs give me a terror of a headache."

Paul is not alone. In fact, the "hot dog headache" is fairly common. Fortunately, Paul had made the connection between his headaches and that particular food (plus a few others). His was a simple solution to a potentially difficult problem.

Possibly a change of diet can alter the frequency of migraines. Altering what you eat is among the changes we refer to as nonspecific treatments. In other words, anyone can try them and most of the time they help, at least a little.

Preventive Nonspecific Treatments

When we were first assessing Joan, we asked her to eliminate certain foods from her diet. Doing so reduced the intensity of her headaches somewhat, but made very little difference in their frequency, so we went on to other things. I suggest you try these changes as a first and simplest attempt to manage your headache.

Altering the Foods You Eat

For those of you who understand chemistry, these are the substances you want to eliminate from your diet: monosodium glutamate, nitrates, nitrites, phenylethylamine, and tyramine. Besides the foods mentioned below, other foods containing some phenylethylamine include dairy products, smoked fish, eggs, tomatoes, and wheat. We usually don't preclude these foods from people's diets, for they supply much-needed nutrients; but you might want to avoid them temporarily during your experiment.

Aged cheeses and yogurt. Most cheeses except the gooey ones that spoil quickly, such as cottage cheese and cream cheese, are aged and therefore contain tyramine as well as phenylethylamine. Sharp cheeses especially do. Processed American cheeses do not; your Velveeta, for example, is okay. Check the label. Most aged cheeses are labelled as such. And forego yogurt.

"What?" you cry. "No Parmesan on my spaghetti or Monterey jack with my tacos?"

That's right, at least for a while. See if it makes a difference.

Alcohol. No beer with your tacos, either. Besides alcohol, beer, champagne, gin, vodka, and red wines also contain tyramine, a substance which can affect blood pressure.

Avocados. "Rats! There goes the guacamole, too. What are you doing to me?"

Cured meats. Bacon, hot dogs, ham, bologna, salami, pepperoni, and summer sausages contain nitrites used in their curing. Some persons react powerfully to nitrites. Migraine is one sort of reaction.

Bananas, broadbean pods, canned figs. "Who in their right mind eats broadbean pods? That's the stuff the prodigal son watched the pigs eat. He couldn't choke it down."

We're just telling you, because most plants contain toxins and other chemicals. Plants are extremely complex chemically, and some of those chemicals hit susceptible humans wrong. Bananas and broadbean pods, but not the broadbeans themselves, contain such chemicals.

Chicken livers. "No love lost there. I can do without." But for some, chicken livers are a favorite food.

Chinese food and any others containing MSG. "Aw, now you're really hitting me where it hurts!"

Monosodium glutamate, abbreviated MSG, is used

to sharpen the flavor of many foods. Check the labels on your seasonings such as Worcestershire sauce, meat tenderizers, Accent, flavor enhancers, steak sauces, dip mixes, some dry soups, and bouillon. Take heart; those restaurants which prepare foods fresh, including Chinese restaurants, will gladly leave out the MSG if you ask them to.

"Yeah, but still, to give up my Chinese food . . ."

It gets worse.

Chocolate. "Not chocolate too! This is like finding out your best friend could be an axe murderer!"

This contains a caffeine-like substance that is a possible migraine trigger. Hang tight!

Citrus fruits and their juices. Citrus includes lemon, lime, limon, grapefruit, and orange. However, apple, cranberry, grape, and pineapple juices are *not* citrus. They're fine. Tomato juice and V8 do not contain citrus, but tomato may have suspicious quantities of phenylethylamine. Use tomato juice with caution, if at all.

Coffee and tea, caffeinated or decaffeinated. Caffeine during a migraine episode sometimes helps. Between episodes, avoid it. But there are other toxins in coffee as well, which is why we ask you to eliminate it entirely. We cannot recommend herb teas as substitutes because they are highly complex chemically, and no two are alike. Herb teas containing the wrong ingredients for you, although they may be perfectly harmless to most people, can really nail you.

Herring, especially pickled herring. It has significant amounts of phenylethylamine. So does chocolate, but I don't hear you howling about pickled herring.

"I like it all right, but it's not critical, you know?"

Nitrates. "I don't eat nitrates."

Actually, you might. For example, hamburger might be treated with nitrates to keep it looking pink and fresh longer. If you are in doubt, ask the butcher or meat counter clerk.

Nuts. Some people are sensitive to nuts, so while you're altering your diet, cut these out also.

Onions. "That's okay. I wasn't going to have tacos anyhow."

Now that you have modified your eating habits, let's look at another part of your life-style—your sleep habits.

Stabilizing Your Eat-and-Sleep Patterns

Bill, a volunteer firefighter, was called out on a structure fire at 11 P.M. Friday night. He got home at 3 A.M. No matter. He's off Saturdays, so he was able to sleep in. He awoke at 9 with a howling headache. It must have been the smoke, right? But then, he occasionally got these headaches, usually on a day off, even when he hadn't been out on a fire. Whatever the cause, Bill felt miserable.

In clinical work, I and others have found that two things which sometimes trigger migraines are more or less related—sleep habits and eating habits. Bill was affected by breaks in his usual patterns of sleep, but they were often unavoidable. He had to go out when called. Fires do not occur at convenient times.

Similarly, if you change your eating habits abruptly, or delay eating, you may get a headache. We suspect hypoglycemia, low blood sugar, is involved here. Blood picks up and distributes the sugar which comes from the foods you eat. If you miss a meal or go on a stringent diet, your blood runs low on sugar because the source of supply has been cut off. If you pig out on a high-sugar treat, delayed hypoglycemia occurs because after the blood is overloaded with sugar, it dumps the sugar resulting in lower than normal blood levels.

Bill had no intention of missing breakfast when he slept in late the next morning; he simply postponed it. So in effect he did indeed miss the meal that should have occurred. That's all his body knew. Your body does not tolerate promises. If it needs sugar, it wants sugar now. "Later, when I get up," won't cut it.

Bill (and you), therefore, can probably reduce his incidence of migraine two ways:

1) Stick to regular patterns of sleeping and eating. Try to take meals at about the same time each day. That way the blood always has some available sugar to haul around.

2) Compensate for irregularities. Bill's normal time of rising on weekdays is 6 A.M. He might have gotten up with the alarm at about 6 A.M., had a glass of fruit juice, and returned to bed for an additional three hours of needed rest. The sugar from the juice would keep his blood system satisfied until he rose at the later hour and ate breakfast.

Examine your sleeping and eating patterns, comparing them to the incidence of headaches. Is there a correlation? What are other extenuating factors? For example, when Bill went out on that fire, he was burning calories like a madman at a time when he normally would be asleep. Calories equal sugar. He was depleting his sugar supply late at night, which compounded the effects of his delayed breakfast.

Now sit down and build yourself a plan for preventing sugar depletion and sugar overload. Follow through on that plan for three or four months at least, depending on the usual frequency of your headaches. See if it doesn't help.

Moderating Exercise

If you suffer migraines, you may find that strenuous exercise, sudden exhausting exercise that your body is not accustomed to, or exercise after eating or smoking may be triggers. Several of my clients noted that they suffered migraines at the beginning of the city amateur soccer season. After a winter of virtual inactivity, all those healthy young men and women got out on the field and ran. And sweated. And wheezed. And didn't really get into shape until about the third week of the playing season. And some of them suffered more than just aching muscles. So establish a regimen of regular moderate exercise for yourself. Walking is excellent. Don't overdo it. Try to walk daily or nearly so. It will almost certainly help.

Nonspecific Treatment During an Episode

Joan is an authority on what won't work for a migraine; she tried just about every folk cure and nonprescription treatment she ever heard of. One was cold. Cold sometimes provides relief.

Cold. There are several ways to deliver cold to your suffering head. One is to use the commercially available ice packs which you either put in the fridge or freezer beforehand or crush at the time you use them. The ones that are warm until you break a small tube inside are handy when travelling or in other circumstances where a refrigerator is not available.

Another way to deliver cold is either an English icebag or a makeshift container for holding ice. If you make yourself an icebag, you'll need something waterproof to hold the ice. A plastic vegetable bag or frozen foods bag serves nicely. Crush the ice, put it in, and seal the bag. But never just place the plastic bag of ice directly against your skin. Put a buffer of some sort between the skin and you. A dish towel will work well. If you hold ice directly against your skin, you may cause frostbite or local freezing. The tissue destruction from a frozen spot can cause real problems.

Companies make ice or "blue ice" pillows or appliances you put on your head. However, cold doesn't work for everyone. If a makeshift ice bag will not work for you, neither will an expensive appliance. Try out cold first before investing much money.

Sleep. Five or six hours of rest and sleep may ease a migraine. Sitting or lying quietly in a dark room usually helps. Low light level and low noise level are key here.

Over-the-counter drugs. Joan tried nearly every over-the-counter drug that promised relief, too. On her pharmacist's advice she tried products containing ibuprofen first, which seems to work as well as anything when the menstrual cycle is involved. Take ibuprofen for seven to ten days, starting about five days before period time. For many women, this regimen will to some degree prevent headaches which are related to the menstrual cycle. To blunt a headache already in progress, try aspirin and caffeine remedies. Check the label for the magic words among the ingredients: ibuprofen or aspirin and caffeine. Always take aspirin and ibuprofen with food—they can cause stomach irritation after long term use.

Folk remedies did not work for Joan, nor did over-the-counter medicines. It was time to tackle the pain big time, and that is when Mark arranged to bring her to the clinic.

Specific Treatment

We were already at work alleviating Joan's migraines during the time that we were exploring and assessing her traits and motivations. She was taking specific medicines to control the pain when a headache struck. The drugs were only partially successful, but she was grateful for any improvement.

Why not simply put Joan on a lifetime medicine regimen, the way certain high blood pressure patients or diabetics do? We don't want to do that because it's dangerous in the long term. Medications, you see, work only with the physical. They alter body chemistry in some way. The body's chemistry is so thoroughly entwined in itself that even medicines with ''no'' side effects have some side effects; they just don't seem to be severe or dangerous. We always prefer to manage headaches without medication. That, however, is not always possible.

If you are under clinical care for migraine, you will probably receive medication to ease the pain, but not always. Some medicines have such strong side effects in certain people that the migraine is actually preferable to the medicine that would ease its effects.

Alleviating the Pain

In the case of a woman in her thirties who suffered excruciating migraine, underlying her symptoms were very strong psychological issues dealing with obsession, false guilt, true guilt, and other problems. From her pastor she obtained some excellent insights and battled her problem for many months. To combat the disabling pain, her family doctor prescribed narcotics, the strongest and most addictive pain medicines available.

While she took the medicine, she could not think clearly or well. Off them, she was climbing the walls with pain. Finally, she came to us for specialized attention for the migraine problem. I put her on Toradol, a new medicine created for pain control. Toradol often relieves migraine pain without the potential for addiction. The Toradol alleviated the pain without knocking her over. She could think. She could function. That intervention permitted her to work on her other issues. Her own hard work, with Toradol, resolved her problem.

Another woman, Thelma, fought frequently with her husband. She suffered severe migraines. She and her husband both knew that they had to work on their marriage problems. When they came to me, the first thing I did was pull her off the handfuls of pills she was taking.

"The medicine I'm prescribing instead," I told her, "is an antidepressant that—"

"But I'm not depressed!" Thelma insisted. "Angry as hornets, yes. Sad, yes. Frustrated, yes. But not depressed."

"That's right," I said. "This antidepressant also has a strong pain relief component. If you're not depressed, it won't cause any psychological problems, and it may help the migraines."

It did. They got to work. And she did great.

I am of the opinion that the better informed the patient is, the better the outcome will be. That is why I always discuss medications with my patients, explaining what the pills do and what the possible effects are. Let me do that for you right here, summarizing the commonly used over-the-counter and prescription medications. Before taking them, however, you should discuss them with your doctor.

Keep in mind that at least two dozen naturally occurring chemicals do different things in your brain, and so does each kind of medication. Medications may help these natural chemicals do their jobs, sometimes working with your brain chemistry, sometimes working against it. So when one type of pill doesn't work well, we often try new or different ones or adjust the dosage. It's okay (in fact, it's expected) for your doctor to say, "Let's change this and try something else."

Nonprescription Products:

Aspirin plus caffeine. People for whom nonprescription medications work seem to find this combination works well. It doesn't prevent much, but it can help the pain and other effects.

Ibuprofen. Advil, Nuprin, and Medipren are some nonprescription ibuprofen products. Ibuprofen appears to work best as a preventative, especially in the case of women whose headaches are tied to menstrual cycles. Try taking the medicine for ten days straight, beginning five days before the expected period.

Prescription Products: Abortive Therapy

Abortive therapy means that as the headache starts, you quickly medicate to try to cut it off early—nip it in the bud, so to speak. This is a particularly nice option for patients who have a little warning that a migraine is coming on. Following are some prescription drugs that perform this function:

Sumatriptan (Imitrex™). This is brand new and shows great promise. Careful tests and studies indicate that it quells all symptoms in half of the patients treated, and it reduced symptoms for nearly three-fourths of the study group. With it, migraine victims can resume at least a part of normal activity, and bright light no longer bothers them as much. It is only given subcutaneously—that is, just beneath the skin—where the body quickly absorbs it. The side effects, such as some tingling, dizziness, warm-hot reactions, and irritation at the injection site, are minor and go away quickly.

Administering Sumatriptan beneath the skin obviously requires a hypodermic needle. Going to the doctor when a migraine strikes not only postpones treatment, it may be impossible for many. So researchers developed a syringe for patients to use themselves by modifying a hypodermic device already used by diabetics. The experiment worked quite well.

Sumatriptan apparently works in two areas: on the suddenly dilated cranial blood vessels and also directly at nerve endings. That means it soothes and helps to relax the nerves. It may also act as a vasoconstrictor.

The ergots. Prior to Sumatriptan, these medicines were the first line of treatment. Ergotamine or ergotamine plus caffeine (Cafergot) are used carefully because they encourage nausea. They also slow down absorption in the stomach, so you might ask about suppositories if the pills are not working well. An ergotamine inhaler is available, but it's expensive.

Ergotamine prevents the blood vessels from expanding rapidly. It's important, therefore, to receive ergotamine as early as possible, especially during an aura (the symptoms before the headache), when the blood vessels are still constricting. They are just about ready to dilate and open, and that's what causes the pain. Ergotamine helps prevent this action.

DHE-45 is a short way of saying dihydroergotamine mesylate. It is usually delivered beneath the skin; that is, you will receive a shot or perhaps intravenous treatment. The IV gets it to your system the fastest, of course. Your doctor will give you something that will first ward off nausea and help your body absorb the DHE-45—probably metoclopramide or prochlorperazine. Then when you take the DHE-45, it goes right to work.

Others. Midrin, a combination of medicines, is usually less nauseating than the ergots. Others sometimes given include Naproxen, one of a class of anti-inflammatory drugs called NSAIDs, pure oxygen, hydroxyzine (an antihistamine), certain steroids, phenothiazines (a group of antipsychotic medicines), or muscle relaxers.

Prescription Drugs: Prophylactic Therapy

Prophylactic therapy, as opposed to abortive therapy, prevents the headache altogether. Prophylactic strategies work great for some people, not at all for others. We usually find ourselves having to shoot for a reduction in the number and severity of migraines rather than a perfect, headache-free cure. Prophylactic treatment is normally required if migraines occur more than twice a month, if the patient simply cannot find relief with medication during an attack, or if an attack lasts over forty-eight hours. The medicine is usually taken continuously.

Beta-adrenergic blockers such as propranolol (Inderal) or nadolol are generally effective (incidentally, pindolol does *not* prevent migraine).

Calcium channel blockers. (Procardia, Calan)

Sodium valproate (Depakene) worked especially well in trials with people suffering *really* severe headaches.

Certain antidepressants: amitriptyline (Elavil) often works even when there's no depression. Dosage varies widely with different people. Antidepressants in low doses are remarkably effective for pain relief. They also may assist in lifting minor symptoms of depression, although this effect is minimal at the low doses usually given for pain control.

Methysergide (Sansert) often triggers severe side effects.

MAO (monoamine-oxidase inhibitors) such as phenelzine (Nardil) require some diet changes, but work 80 percent of the time, often when nothing else does.

Again I emphasize that no single drug is a miracle

cure. You cannot pop a pill and solve your migraine problem. Sorry. The pill is only to shunt aside the distraction of the headache itself, enabling you to work efficiently. And believe me, much work is required to find the root cause of your headache and then effect the life-style changes and the changes in thinking that will resolve the problem. But that's the only way. And it's worth it!

Some Available Drugs

Non-prescription (Over-the-counter)

Aspirin, salycilates
Ibuprofens
Acetaminophens

Prescription Drugs

Narcotics (controlled substances requiring a special type of prescription)
  codeine
  morphine
  Demerol
  percodan
  vicodin
  Dilantid
Ergotamines
Ergotamines plus caffeine
Antidepressants
Beta blockers
Prednisone
Sumatriptan
Minor tranquilizers
Combination medicines

Rooting Out and Treating the Hidden Causes

We have already discussed Joan's sense of self-worth. Now I established a plan with Joan to help her make herself feel better. First, I asked her to memorize some verses from Scripture in order to tackle her guilt. Joan was not a strong Christian, but she respected the faith enough to try it.

God's word speaks powerfully! Joan had never realized that God does not weigh your worth by what you do. It opened a whole new horizon to her.

Consider David, the shepherd who became king. He was a womanizer who erred grievously with Bathsheba, committing adultery and murder. He made serious mistakes when he heard his son Absalom was killed, when he numbered Israel, and at other times. If God worked on a point system, David would have been dead meat. God does not, and David, despite his flaws, remained the apple of God's eye. David never let his imperfect life stop him from enthusiastically loving and trusting his Lord.

Nothing takes the place of reading and memorizing Scripture. I recommend it in the strongest terms. When you fill your mind and heart with God's messages to you, false messages fade to the background. Use a commentary or topical Bible to choose verses. But do, like Joan, let God speak to you about His love for you. (I also often recommend a book by Dr. Larry Stephens of our clinic titled *Please Let Me Know You, God*. His book helps each of us to see our loving God more clearly.)

Joan might be on the move constantly, but her physical activity was like a jackrabbit—run, run, run or sit. She did little in between. I prescribed for her a moderate exercise program that involved walking on a regular basis. She paid renewed attention to diet and sleep patterns.

Joan came in, too, for counseling every week to talk out her problems. As her insight into her inner thoughts increased, she was able to make healthy changes in her thinking. You may choose to use a counselor for this important step. If you wish to work on it on your own, enlist the ears and heart of a trusted friend. If that trusted friend is also a migraineur, you can perhaps listen to each other. Talk about problems. Explore insights. Try to help each other see how and why you think as you do. Where are there control trouble spots? How about low self-worth trouble spots? Guilt? Anxiety? Anger?

Repressed anger so often erupts as a headache.

"But I'm not angry!" you insist.

Okay, you're not angry. Now sit down with your trusted friend, or in front of a mirror if need be, and explore this issue.

Could you be angry at God? My good friend Paul Meier claims, "I get mad at God once or twice a week because I'm stupid." Paul is not stupid, of course. He's one of the most unstupid people I've ever known. He was referring, rather, to his knee-jerk reaction of questioning God's sovereignty ("Why, oh why, is this happening to me?") and not going with God's flow. Everyone does it. The people who refuse to acknowledge they are doing it are suppressing anger.

Are you mad at others or mad at yourself down deep, where it doesn't show? In our hospital practice—and I mean all of us at Minirth Meier New Life

Clinics, with thousands of patients—we see that the nicest, most conscientious people are the ones with the worst headaches. They're nice because they want to be. They strive to be. People who blow up and get ugly aren't nice in their own eyes, and so they stuff their anger. Believe me, that anger is going to express itself somehow.

Some physical problems turn out to be caused by sins we don't know we're committing. Examples are holding grudges, planning or working vengeance, engaging in willful sin and refusing to acknowledge it (as David did with Bathsheba, for instance), selfish fancies, unjustly controlling others. A lot of emotional pain comes out of sin when the Holy Spirit is convicting a Christian and that person refuses to repent. David didn't deal with his sin at first, and when he kept silent, he had a terrible pain inside.

Very often I find unresolved and displaced anxiety in my clients. When those issues are resolved, the headaches usually fade or cease altogether. Not always, but usually.

Grieving is involved here in this stage of treatment. Much has been lost to these migraines—lost time, lost relationships, lost productivity, lost comfort. In their place came confusion, anger, anxiety. All these losses must be recognized and grieved. This grief process is an important way in which you deal with the problems you found.

Slowly, Joan's thinking changed. As she came to grips with her need to achieve and replaced it with the sure knowledge that God loves her as she is, the headaches faded. Mark avowed his love for her—not her accomplishments but her. Joan understood that any accomplishments and goals attained were mere icing on the cake.

His support helped Joan greatly. If a friend or relative of yours suffers migraine, your support can similarly help them. Make it available and make it generous.

Now I want to proffer the advice I give clients constantly. You've heard it all before, every bit of it. But now I'm asking you to apply it to headache management. I'm asking you to alter your thinking, your deepest way of looking at things, to better relieve the stresses that bring on discomfort. These points will not help every migraine sufferer, but they help most if they are properly taken to heart and put into action.

Remember that logic does nothing for emotions. Logic and emotion are not on the same wavelength; they're not even centered in the same parts of the brain. We're talking not about logic here but about facts you incorporate into your heart to the extent that they change the way you think. The way you think then changes your life-style to some degree—your outlook, at the very least.

Heart Knowledge

This process will work differently for every person because every person is different. Do these points speak to you?

Be verbal. Say what you think. Certainly you should be judicious. Certainly you should season your words. But don't stifle your feelings. Your feelings are every bit as valuable as anyone else's and deserve nurturing and expression. Clear the air.

You don't need the approval of everyone. It would be very nice to be loved by all but that will never happen, no matter how lovable you try to make yourself.

This point really came home to May. May spent her whole life in a small Texas town near the Arkansas border. She knew the power of gossip and innuendo. She knew she would never live anywhere else. She therefore had convinced herself that she must win everyone's admiration and favor constantly or she would be ostracized. She saw things as white or black. Because of a combination of factors in her early life, she could not see a middle ground: gray.

May discovered that her migraines seemed to come on when someone criticized her or spoke ill of her. When she realized how completely she was letting other people control her health and comfort and when she finally grasped that it was absolutely impossible to please everyone 100 percent of the time, the migraines nearly disappeared. Just becoming aware of these deep seated misbeliefs did not do the trick. Changing her thinking and life-style did.

May's sister Janelle suffered migraines also. When May found relief, she sent her sister to me. Janelle had another life-changing discovery to make:

I am not worthless just because someone important to me doesn't like me. Neither May nor Janelle had a warm relationship with their father. He was a hard man, bitter and disappointed by life, who saw nothing good in raising daughters. He never abused them physically or even yelled at them, but they got the message loud and clear: "You should have been boys. You should have been better."

Janelle had an extremely difficult time working past her father's callous disregard. Janelle especially benefited from the memorization of Scripture. She needed a constant outpouring of messages that God does truly love her, that she is indeed an important child of His.

Sad to say, Janelle has not yet mastered her headaches. She has not fully converted her head knowledge into heart knowledge, but she's working on it and it's getting better. The headaches do not come as often anymore.

The migraineur will be quick to tell you that any improvement is a blessing.

Be mature, not perfect. Maturity, you have often heard, is a journey, not a destination. Perfection is not an attainable goal, but it is a worthy one. I find I must often counsel clients in those basic precepts. I find, too, that the clients usually already knew that but were disregarding it. In essence we took that knowledge off the back burner and put it right up front.

You can succeed but not in every little endeavor. This was the message Joan needed to take to heart. She excelled. But she felt, down deep that she had to excel constantly. She had to learn that it's okay to flub something. Joan still has trouble with the concept, but she has learned to laugh off the goof-ups.

To ask for help is not to admit defeat. Men in particular, being trained from infancy to be self-sufficient, have a hard time with this one. Two exercises I find helpful to overcome this mind-set are:

1) to research ways in which historically prominent people received significant help (hint: they all did; Columbus from Queen Isabella, for instance), and

2) to study Scripture on the subject. David received both Michal's and Jonathan's help to escape Saul's clutches—and they were Saul's children! An angel gave Peter his get out of jail free card in Acts 12:6–11. Regardless of the human help available, God was there in every instance; God is there for the migraineur too.

As you deal with your migraine (or as your loved one does), do not hesitate to ask for help from people around you. Also, pay attention to opportunities to be of help. The paralyzing thought of the migraineur is "God can't use me when I'm like this!" Self-image plummets when a migraine bears down. Certainly He can use you! If He used Balaam's donkey, He can use you, even when you're incapacitated with one of those headaches.

"Yes," you reply grimly, "but Balaam's donkey didn't have a migraine."

Think positively. A negative attitude is typical, and no wonder. The migraineur feels not only overwhelmed but defeated. Those negative feelings themselves can cause a problem. If you continue with obsessively negative thinking, that in itself can trigger a headache.

Suggesting these attitudes and steps is easy. Making them so much a part of you that they alter your life-style is not. In fact, for some migraineurs it is literally impossible. The person in the throes of one of those headaches cannot think at all. Hanging over that person constantly is the nagging dread at the back of the mind, "There will be another. When will the next one strike?" Will your plans be scuttled by an untimely migraine? A vacation spoiled? A special event—a wedding or birthday, perhaps—marred? Will you be able to function at work?

If introspection and self-help do not do the trick, it is time to seek professional help. Sometimes over-the-counter pain medications suffice. When they do not, a visit to the doctor is definitely in order.

Children and Migraine

Do kids get these headaches? They certainly do. The vast majority of afflicted children have a family history of migraine. Part of the problem might be observation within the family. Especially for young children, that is the only way they learn what words and concepts mean. They see Mom or Dad with the monstrous headache. That must be what "sick" is. That must be how one garners attention. I do not mean to suggest that a child consciously considers these things. The thoughts and feelings run much deeper, on a subconscious level, strong enough to cause migraines.

But the migraines are real, not figments of a child's imagination. In fact, they happen even more frequently in migraine-prone kids than in adults. Often, children feel they are being punished somehow, that they are victims. That's certainly to be expected; Joan felt exactly the same way.

You can tell a child is afflicted by the actions you see—holding the head, acting listless and irritable, vomiting. Fever and loss of appetite may also occur.

"But kids do that constantly," you protest. "You know children. They act irritable if you so much as look at them cross-eyed. And kids miss no little opportunity to throw up. And when they whine, 'I hurt,' you have no idea what it means."

True. Your first clue, other than those signs, is that Mom or Dad is also a migraineur. Over half of kids with migraines have parents who are afflicted similarly.

Obviously we don't want to pump high-powered medicines into a child. Dietary control seems to work as well as anything for child migraineurs. Try to keep bedtimes and mealtimes regular. Set aside a specific time for schoolwork and provide snacks. Where are the child's stress and tension points? Can you reduce them? In those very rare cases of out of control headaches in a child, your doctor may want to try preventing episodes with specific medicines.

Mark and Joan did not have children but they wanted kids. However, Joan wanted to bring her migraines under control first. How could she care for an infant or toddler if she was incapacitated?

While Joan was working on her problem, Mark had one of his own. His headaches did not resemble hers because they arose from a different source. Let's look next at how the slings and arrows of outrageous fortune can generate a doozy of a brain-wringer—the tension headache.

CHAPTER 6

Tension Headaches: Symptoms and Causes

For me, it's driving in the snow." Kate, from Northern Michigan, talks about what causes tension for her. "It's not that I can't do it. I can. I've been doing it for years. But I just hate it. My trapezius muscles all bunch up here; they really tie themselves into knots." She lays her hands on the triangular muscles between the back of her neck and the back of her shoulders. "And I get really stiff from the constant tension."

"I hate driving in snow, too," says her friend Alice. "My muscles don't knot up, but boy, do I get a killer headache."

Killer headache. Oh, how the advertisements for aspirin and other painkillers love to dramatize your headache! "When you haven't got time for the pain . . ." When *do* you? I remember long ago in a TV ad, a very important-looking fellow would stand next to a highly stylized chart of a person with a highly stylized gastrointestinal tract, and point to all the little As swirling around down inside there. Then little Bs would stream purposefully through the system. Anyone could see that those little Bs were going to make short work of the headache while the As were still stumbling around, bumping into each other and causing stomach upset.

Americans will lay down about $500,000,000 this year on over-the-counter painkillers, and most will be purchased for headaches. Most of the headaches for which those painkillers will be purchased will be tension headaches, the headaches dramatized with so much flair on TV.

There are reasons that advertisers dwell so heavily on tension headaches. For one thing, migraines usually do not respond well to over-the-counter medications. You don't want to advertise your product as a cure for something it won't cure. Then your customer won't buy your product for the things it will alleviate, and that's the other reason. Tension headaches usually respond to easily-obtained remedies.

Also, most people get tension headaches now and then which are typically related to muscle tension associated with stress and anxiety.

But not necessarily for the same reasons. One man's meat is another man's poison. The two ladies above who were talking about driving in Michigan snow illustrate that. Neither likes to. One gets all tensed up. The other gets a headache. Actually, although the second woman's muscles don't knot up, they are tensing as well, and they are generating, or helping to generate, her headaches.

"Okay," you say. "Since tension headaches respond to medication, I pop a couple of pills. No big thing."

Tension headaches are indeed a big thing in several ways. For one, they signal that something is not right. Tension headaches, while very *common*, are not *nor-*

mal. If you remove their cause, you've improved your health and probably your outlook on life. That's worth a lot! And being pain free is a whole lot better than trying to beat down the pain with pills. Even if pills alleviate the pain, there's still the sodden, dull feeling they leave with you. You can relieve a tension headache, but you sometimes cannot completely dispel it. Also, migraine sufferers know that a tension headache can escalate into a migraine; they have a vested interest in avoiding tension headaches at almost any cost.

Mark's tension headaches did not escalate beyond annoyance, but they annoyed him immensely. He had trouble finding medications that would dull the pain. He wanted a cure almost as much as Joan did.

We first explored possible causes beyond the obvious ones, trying to reveal the headache triggers. Remember that there are usually several causes. You can't come up with just one and be certain you've found them all.

Causes

Stress

How would you rate the following activities as stressors? Stress to the max? So-so stress? No big deal?

1. ___ Caring for a toddler younger than age two
2. ___ Caring for two children under the age of two
3. ___ Working in a day-care center
4. ___ Foregoing coffee breaks to complete a rush job

5. ___ Getting three or more gotta-have-it-yesterday rush jobs in a week
6. ___ Learning that your supervisor expects more from you than you're capable of delivering
7. ___ Technical rock climbing in Yosemite
8. ___ Hang gliding
9. ___ Being first on the scene of a suicide or major accident
10. ___ Camping along a creek in Arkansas when it's pouring rain

I would rate number 10 "No stress at all." I love camping, and if it's raining, so what? You string up a tarp back-to-the-wind and build a cheery fire and sing songs as you make s'mores. My wife, Mary Alice, however, might rate number 10 pretty high. She enjoys camping, but only to a point.

In short, different people would rate those items in different ways; I mean, very widely different. Fine people volunteer for numbers 3 and 9 because they see it as work to be done and they don't mind doing it; for them the stress is minimal. Many people use numbers 7 and 8 for stress *relief!* I must never listen to things I might consider stressors in a patient's life and assume they affect the patient the same way they would affect me.

Now build a list that is all your own. What are the big stressors in your life? Do they relate to job? Family? Relationships? Things you must do that you hate? Things you fear? Most people can cite a dozen or more irritants that apply stress in their lives. If you are subject to tension headaches, stress points may well be triggers, especially if several occur close together.

Like the camel carrying straw, each of us has a load limit.

Anxiety and Depression

I suppose we could call these factors stressors also. They certainly are in their own way. There is a strong correlation between headache, anxiety, and depression.

For Kate, both the physical activity of driving in snow and the anxiety that accompanied it contributed to her tenseness. Muscles do nothing unless nerves trigger them. Therefore, any muscle reaction is necessarily a nerve reaction. For Alice, the anxiety plus the physical tension translated into headache. What tends to make you feel anxious? Again, spend some time building a list.

Whether the immediate problem is physical stress, anxiety, or the constant weight of depression, the underlying mechanism, most doctors believe, is the prolonged excessive contraction of posterior neck muscles. These are the muscles Kate was talking about. When they tense up in a stressful situation and stay that way, they reduce circulation in the back of the head immediately above them. The reduced circulation triggers the pain.

"Wait a minute." Mark frowned. "Just exactly what are anxiety and depression? I mean, how do I know whether I have them or not? Is this one of those things where if you have to ask if you have it, you don't have it?"

Excellent question. Anxiety and depression are two things everybody talks about but never explains. Let's define *anxiety* from a medical viewpoint.

Anxiety is fear without an object. The person feels intensely fearful but doesn't know quite why. (In contrast, if a Doberman is chasing you, you feel just as fearful, but you know exactly why.) A low-grade chronic anxiety can rumble along beneath the surface, gnawing at you, eluding your scrutiny. You think it's silly for you to feel so afraid when there's nothing to be afraid of, but it's there. And that doubt about yourself and your feelings further fuels the anxiety. That undercurrent of anxiety can sometimes erupt into an acute anxiety attack.

In contrast to anxiety, depression does not attack; it sneaks in, burrows under. You may not be aware it exists at first. Depression drags out over days or months. The person experiencing depression will feel some of these following nine symptoms every day:

1. A depressed mood, the blues, the blahs.
2. A markedly diminished interest or pleasure in most activities. Things you used to enjoy don't mean much anymore. This includes sex, dining out, sports, games, leisure activities, the job, even the kids.
3. Significant weight loss or gain even though you are not dieting. "Yeah, sure," you grumble, "and with my luck it will be the one I *don't* want. If I'm overweight, I'll gain more, right?"
   Did I mention pessimism?
4. Insomnia or hypersomnia; that is, inability to sleep or too much sleep. Early morning awakenings, 3 or 4 A.M., are a classic sign.
5. Physical slowness or hyperactivity. Do you turn into a fidgeter or a vegetable?

6. Fatigue or loss of energy
7. Feeling of worthlessness, excessive guilt, inappropriate guilt; a woe-is-me attitude taken to extreme
8. Diminished ability to think, to concentrate, to make decisions. Not only are you unable to function well mentally, you don't even want to anymore. It doesn't matter.
9. Recurrent thoughts of death though not fear of dying. This might even be an obsession with death. Usually, recurrent suicidal thoughts go along with it. You may or may not consider an actual suicide plan.

I went over each item with Mark as he explored his thoughts. Although Joan's problem got him down in the dumps, depression in a lasting sense was not a part of his picture. It was as though his headaches generated a mild temporary depression, not the other way around. He lacked most of the symptoms listed above. It may only take a few of the symptoms listed to cause or complicate a headache.

There is indeed another problem which complicates the picture. We are finding that as depression triggers headaches, headaches in turn trigger depression and even feelings of self-hatred. When headache patients under a doctor's care were quizzed, only 55 percent thought their doctor actually understood their problem. They felt consumed by feelings of despair, hopelessness, and isolation when it appeared that they could not control their headaches as well as other people seem to. "There must be something wrong with me! Obviously I'm not trying hard enough. I'm no good, or I could lick this thing."

And society itself doesn't help. How much respect does a headache get in the scheme of things, as compared to, for example, a broken arm? Easy answer. The arm gets lots of sympathy and autographs on its cast. The headache isn't even considered a valid problem.

Stress and anxiety or depression are two causes of tension headaches; foods and medicines are another.

Foods and Medicines

Here is another situation of every person responding differently. In this case, "One man's food is another's poison" is quite literal. Go down the list of foods that can be causes of migraine, in chapter three. They are also associated with tension headaches. Nitrates and nitrites can be particularly insidious villains. A few people are so sensitive to nitrites that a small dose as a food additive can send them to the hospital. They report headache as a major symptom. People with much less sensitivity may still experience headaches when they ingest nitrites. Nitrates usually do not affect you directly, but they turn into nitrites after digestion.

When health magazines first started beating the drum hard about the nasty effects of caffeine, Mark switched to decaf coffee in the mornings. He expected to feel much better.

Mark wagged his head disbelievingly as he told me about it. "I swear, the switch almost killed me! I would have had to get better to die. I was popping aspirin, Tylenol, even those pills women take for cramps during their period. I must really have been addicted to caffeine!"

Going off caffeine suddenly very often causes intense headaches. Once the body becomes accustomed to caffeine, cutting off the supply can wreak havoc. If you're going to reduce your caffeine intake, wean yourself slowly, step by gentle step, over a period of a week or two. Don't go cold turkey.

Eating foods containing tyramine or MSG can cause headaches in some people. If they seem to be a culprit for you, go over that list in chapter three carefully. Some things are worth avoiding.

Drugs that can provoke headache include nitroglycerine (which certain heart patients use to relieve chest pain), high blood pressure pills, certain steroids, certain types of ear drops, and treatments for diabetes such as insulin and oral pills. Some monoamine oxidase inhibitors (a type of antidepressant medicine) can adversely affect people as well, especially if combined with foods containing tyramine.

Other Possible Triggers

Mark grimaced as he showed me the lists he was making. "Look at all this! And I'm supposed to examine all these factors in my life."

"That's right."

"Hmph. I'd say that the only way to avoid a headache is stay home with the curtains drawn, but I suppose even that could trigger one." His sarcasm has some basis in fact. A lot of mundane things you do might be causing headaches.

Add these to the list of possible triggers that you ought to examine closely in your own life:

Excessive eating. This is a specialized instance of a generalized situation we could call "overstressing the body." Taking a heavy load of food on board forces a lot of interlocked body systems into overdrive all at once. Most of these systems are closely associated with the circulatory system. Particularly as we get older and our physiology becomes less flexible, the body may have trouble handling sudden overloads.

Drinking alcohol. Separately from the hangover, a headache in a class all by itself, taking in alcohol can cause chemical changes in your body that trigger headaches. When you examine this possibility, don't think "excessive alcohol?" Think "any alcohol at all?"

Eyestrain, often from prolonged sun glare. This is a specialized case of the general situation of muscles tensing up for long periods of time, akin to Kate's dread of driving in snow.

Low blood sugar. Perhaps the situation doesn't develop enough to trigger a migraine, but it causes enough stress to generate a tension headache. Fortunately, blood sugar level is something you can adjust quite quickly. Almost immediately as you take in sugar, it absorbs into the blood stream through the lining of the mouth and upper digestive tract. Nibbling a naturally sweet food such as fruit or fruit juice, or an unnaturally sweet food such as a candy bar, can alleviate the low blood sugar problem.

Menstrual and other hormonal changes. For years, too many doctors have been telling women, "It's just something you have to put up with." Don't you believe it! On a calendar or in a journal, track your headache symptoms on a scale of one to ten each day in relation to your periods. Do you find yourself more easily angered or saddened at certain times of the month? Certain hormones may be ebbing at those times.

Every couple fights on some occasion; if you are married, do those fights seem to occur most frequently just before menstruation? Now don't assess blame here. One of my clients said, "Well, come to think of it, yes. But it was his fault!" And she proceeded to explain why it was that her husband had initiated the fight. And he did, but her low hormone level escalated the situation to the point of a fight. He did the same things at other times of the month, and she let them go.

Women whose periods have ceased might want to keep track of headaches the way they used to mark the calendar on the first day of periods. Sometimes the headaches take over, so to speak, where the periods left off and continue the pattern the menstrual periods used to follow. The body is trying to follow its usual menstrual cycle, but that cycle has ceased. A headache results instead of a period.

Allergic reactions. The person who doesn't suffer in ragweed season or on other high-pollen days can't begin to imagine the misery of the person who does. Like the old Chinese water torture, the constant draining of sinuses, the constant irritation of itchy eyes and sneezing, the constant . . . you get the idea. Headaches result in two ways. One is the body's physiological responses and the other is the annoyance, which causes tension and thereby causes the same kind of headache our two snow-drivers were talking about.

All these possible triggers and others are due to fairly common body responses that have somehow gone awry. Possibly, by understanding how the body functions under mundane conditions, you can find the special conditions that are causing you problems.

Your Body's Chemical Processing Plant

Let's look at your specific situation. Picture your body as a big chemical plant. Every thing you do and every thought you think takes energy. Even sleeping requires energy. All that energy, as well as every thought and movement you make, is created by chemical reactions at the tips of nerves, in your digestive system, in each cell—all over.

Think about a typical day that is headache free. Let's call this your chemical baseline. This is what your body does when it's not encountering unusual or difficult conditions.

Now think about any conditions that would alter the body's usual chemical activity. Those conditions might trigger a headache.

Some doctors feel that cranial artery dilation (probably the body's knee-jerk reaction to restricted blood flow from muscle tenseness nearby) is the underlying mechanism. That is, when blood vessels in the head enlarge, headaches result. Other doctors believe that the cause arises first in the nerves of the head and the blood vessels are merely responding to the nerve stimulae. Whether either or both theories are correct, we know there is a nerve component (as when emotion or stress triggers an attack) together with a fluid pressure component.

A word you ought to know here is *perfusion*. You are aware that every cell in your body receives its oxygen from the blood and dumps its waste products into the blood. Lungs replace the oxygen and get rid of some waste—the carbon dioxide—and kidneys filter out other wastes. All this occurs as blood cells—corpuscles—crowd their way through capillaries.

The capillaries, extending absolutely everywhere through body tissues, are tiny vessels only one blood corpuscle wide. The body cell abutting against the capillary seizes oxygen as the corpuscle slides by, snatching it right in through the capillary wall. The cell shoves its waste out through the capillary wall, where the blood corpuscles and fluids pick it up and carry it away to be disposed of. It all happens in an instant! Amazing!

That exchange of oxygen and waste chemicals is perfusion. If blood pressure drops, perfusion suffers; the cells cannot snatch their oxygen and dump their wastes as well. In fact, perfusion suffers (for different reasons) if pressure builds too high too. When perfusion in the head is curtailed, headache usually results. If perfusion in the head is *really* curtailed, the patient either faints or goes into traumatic shock.

In the brain, oxygen and wastes absolutely must be delivered and delivered well to the right places, all the time. So when your doctor talks about lack of good perfusion for one reason or another, that's what he's talking about—a lack of prompt delivery. It is a major underlying cause of headache.

Signs and Symptoms

Mark grimaced. "Signs and symptoms of a tension headache? Everyone knows them!" Mark had reason to feel a little testy. Joan had been driven to her knees by another of her headaches. Her condition actually represented progress. Previously she had been knocked off her feet. Still, the pressure had given Mark another of his increasingly frequent tension headaches.

Tension headaches are episodic. That is, they happen when they happen, not usually in specific patterns like migraines. They can occur daily or rarely, morning or evening. Often they start slow in the morning and build through the day as pressure piles upon pressure. People experiencing chronic headaches can suffer headache pain almost daily, for weeks, or even years.

Tension headaches are normally bilateral: they occur on both sides of the head. Often they start at the back of the head as a dull tightness. The pain usually does not pulsate. Rather it gnaws on you as a steady, grinding pain at either the back or the front of the head.

"Yeah, that's me," Mark affirmed. "And when it really gets cooking I feel blah; I mean *very* blah. I can't concentrate. At work I have to assign myself donkey tasks; you know, stuff you don't have to think about as you do it, mindless stuff. I can't think clearly."

"Do you ever experience dizziness or body aches?" I asked.

"No."

Some folks do. But almost never do bright lights and loud noises pose a problem as they so often do for migraine sufferers. Tipping the head quickly or moving quickly does not seem to aggravate the condition. You can go up and down stairs, for instance, without feeling a whole lot worse. Like Mark, most tension headache victims find their problem inhibits but does not prohibit their functioning.

Keep in mind as you analyze your own symptoms that a patient is not limited to one type of headache to the exclusion of all others. Migraine and tension may represent two ends of a scale, but both types may occur in the same person. Still, because they differ we must treat each separately.

What Else to Watch For

Like most headache patients, Mark harbored some very real worries down deep. What if this is one of those horror stories you hear about where the guy thinks it's an ordinary headache and it turns out to be a tumor the size of a volleyball? he wondered. What if you think you're fine and suddenly you drop over dead? And then there's that word *cancer.*

One of the first steps we always take when evaluating headaches is to rule out malignancies and other problems.

Here is a list of some of the characteristics of serious conditions that might seem at first like a simple tension headache:

- Tumors cause pressure which can cause pain. The pain usually starts on the same side of your head as the tumor and then generalizes—that is, spreads and diffuses—as the tumor grows. Nerve and muscle problems usually accompany pain and pressure in this scenario.
- Brain abscess, a pocket of infection, may cause a sudden stunning headache, an unusual headache you never had before.

- Blood vessel abnormalities, present from birth, such as aneurisms may cause pain. An aneurism is a weak spot in a vessel that balloons out and stretches. Like a toy balloon, it can rupture if the weakness and blood pressure are sufficient.
- Subdural hematomas are nearly always preceded by headaches. A subdural hematoma is a pocket of fresh blood within the membranes that cover the brain, usually caused by a blow or other injury.
- Infection in the brain and spinal column, such as meningitis or encephalitis, causes a headache to build gradually over a period of hours or days, usually associated with weakness and fever.
- Extremely severe pain around the eye or deep in the eye socket may signal glaucoma, especially if the eye is also red.

Let me recommend, therefore, that you call a doctor if:

- Your headache is accompanied by fever, or other physical symptoms.
- It is the result of a recent head injury, or you lose consciousness.
- It causes drowsiness, particularly if a bump or other injury is involved.
- You experience nausea, vomiting, muscle weakness, tingling, or paralysis.
- You feel pain in one eye or your vision is blurred.
- Pain or tenderness around your eyes and cheekbones worsens when you lean forward and your head feels "full."
- You have high blood pressure.

Headaches may have no relation whatsoever to another serious medical problem. Only one-third of people with brain tumors, for example, report a headache as one of their symptoms. Don't let the presence or absence of headache either panic you or lull you into a false sense of security.

The statistics were all in Mark's favor: far fewer than one in a hundred headaches involve a serious organic condition. By means of a medical workup we determined that Mark had no threatening conditions. His headache was merely that—a headache.

Mark sounded a bit impatient as he said, "This is all very well and good. Now let's get rid of my tension headaches, okay?"

He had done his homework well. He already knew about the strain and tension his wife's headaches caused him. He knew now that some foods may be causing a problem. He had examined most possible stressors as they applied to his personal life-style. Now was the time to do something with what he learned.

Now is the time for you to do something about what you've learned.

CHAPTER 7

Tension Headaches: Treatment

Mark didn't have much confidence that we could ease his headaches. "Look," he insisted, "they're in my head. When Joan gets sick, I feel bad from the worry and stress. You can't change that. You can't do anything about the long checkout lines in the grocery store or the heavy traffic that bugs me. It's hopeless."

To which I replied, "No, I can't change your circumstances. Do you know what the fire triangle is?"

"Yes, I think so. We learned about that in grade school during fire prevention week every year. A fire needs three things in order to burn. Is that it?"

"That's it."

"It needs air—oxygen—and fuel and high temperature. Take away any of the three, and a fire can't burn."

"Exactly. A tension headache requires a trigger, such as stress. That's one leg. The others are nerve irritation and vasodilation. Take away any of the three, and you'll get relief. But in the fire triangle, all three sides are equally important. With a headache, get rid of the trigger and you get rid of the headache. The other two components are secondary. Want to try?"

Mark shrugged. "Let's try."

Removing the Stress

Removing the stress itself is by far the best way to ease tension headaches because it requires no medication. You can't alter the circumstance, but you can alter your reaction to it. Basically, it's attitude adjustment. Mark cannot do a thing about Joan's problem or about driving through the snow, but he can change his attitude toward them.

This is the hardest part, and it reaps the richest return. It involves developing entirely new behavior and thought patterns.

I told Mark about a lady in our clinic who had suffered headaches for years. She was a financial institution manager, very successful and busy, so she figured headaches came with the territory. Eventually her medications weren't touching the pain, and she came to us.

"I'll try to 'tune-up' your meds," I told her, "but you have to change your life-style."

She almost walked out. But she didn't get to the top in her career by doing foolish things, and that would have been silly. She stayed.

"Your behavior," I explained, "has to be truly new, a complete restructuring. We'll program in more relaxation . . ."

"Isn't that a contradiction in terms?" she interrupted. "To program leisure?"

"Not at all. How often do you really kick back and relax?"

"Okay, I'll confess, almost never."

"Right. So we schedule relaxation times. What we're doing, fundamentally, is using a device that is natural to you—scheduling and keeping appointments—and applying it in a new way. This rescheduling wouldn't work well for the person who doesn't watch the clock and doesn't work on a tight appointment schedule. It should work very well for you, however."

As a rule, I recommend that people plan about 80 percent of their day and leave 20 percent unplanned. No appointments, no calls to make, no things to get done. Now and then something will fall into that unplanned space and mess it up. But the wise planner will try to keep it inviolate.

I myself use this eighty-twenty rule. Also, I schedule in times to relax; I'm an inveterate workaholic if I don't keep that kind of tight control on my schedule. Programming in the free time is the only way I can get any. It is so important to relax!

No schedule is so hectic that it can't be adjusted to allow for the really important matters of life. Relaxation is not an option. It is vitally important.

I continued, "Your behavior changes must also include appropriate exercise and more appropriate releases for anger and frustration."

She frowned at me. "Why did you say that?"

"Say what?"

" 'Releases for anger.' How did you know?"

She was so afraid of being referred to as an angry woman, she kept a nice, pleasant, nonconfrontational face to the world, always. Rather than be openly assertive, she managed anger by manipulation and sheer brains, reading people and anticipating what they would do. For her own sake she had to devise some way to express her negative emotions as well as her positive feelings.

People who are truly passive have an even harder time. They don't speak up when they ought to. They let others take unfair advantage in major ways. The anger boils (unfairness always generates anger), and they shove it aside.

"And schedule in some humor, if you can't find it in your workplace," I suggested. Humor is a wonderful healing mechanism, and it's often disregarded. Believe it or not, it generates the same positive changes in brain chemistry that certain pain relievers do.

Having just returned from a business trip to Europe, she scheduled into her week the five hours needed to read Mark Twain's *Innocents Abroad*. She had some time left over, and so on the advice of her assistant manager, she tried Dave Barry's delightfully outlandish travel book. They were different sorts of humor from different eras and different perspectives. Both made her laugh.

This woman had spent her whole life in a headlong charge toward perfection and success. It took her a long time to change gears completely. She stumbled. She blew it often. But with time she blew it only occasionally. The behavior changes replaced her need for medication. She doesn't take anything anymore, and while she's not headache-free, she finds she can live with her occasional mild discomforts.

While Joan was skeptical about the healing power of Scripture, Mark's faith in Christ enabled him to accept my suggestion that meditating on Scripture would give him a better perspective on life and, in turn, might help reduce his headaches. I pointed out some verses that he might memorize so that he could call them up when he needed them.

Which ones should you memorize? I can't tell you. A verse that strikes me as immensely important may not be the most important to your. I suggest you go through the whole book of Proverbs, whether you are a Christian or not. Meditate both on what it says and on the symbolic meanings its nuggets convey. Choose one or two that especially speak to you. Memorize them. Now go through it again. What else speaks to you?

Similarly, study the Psalms. These are the texts of songs that once were sung—and in some cases, they still are. Nearly every one of them sings praise to God. Which one speaks especially to you? Memorize it. Spoken speech and sung speech come from different sources in the brain. Some of my patients who are musically inclined find great fun and help in setting favorite psalms to their own music or poetic rhythms. Try that if you like. Try anything that will make the Scriptures a comfortable, living part of your life.

A friend of mine uses this device to alter his reactions to circumstances: A hundred years from now, who's going to care? "Actually," he says, grinning, "I can just as easily say 'Who's going to care ten years from now? Or one year?' It's my way of prioritizing life." Who will care if he's ten minutes late for an appointment because traffic is especially heavy? Who will care if his boss just erupted in a tantrum punctuated by "This has to be done *now!*"

Essentially, my friend has learned to stop and smell

the flowers, although there are no flowers or fragrance involved. What device can you dream up to help you remember that very few things are essential, and quite probably your headache trigger is not one of them?

People who study how the brain functions have learned that discussion—"mere" words—and behavior changes can alter brain chemistry exactly as do certain drugs, and vice versa. To illustrate, I have a patient named Sam, who was compulsive about yard work. He wanted his lawn and flower beds picture perfect all 365 days of the year. His wife swore that if he preceded her to the grave she was going to bury his lawn mower with him and engrave the fact on his tombstone. Anything that went wrong with Sam's perfect yard stressed him out. Wet weather prevented mowing on schedule, or roto-tilling; bam! Headache. A pesky mole invaded, raising mountains and tunnelling through the lawn and flowers. When over a period of two weeks Sam failed to poison or trap the destructive critter, that little five-inch-long animal literally sent Sam into a tizzy with a debilitating tension headache.

Sam's wife brought him to me for the compulsion, not for the headache. She reasoned, correctly, that if the compulsive behavior were modified, the headaches would fade as well.

With Sam's thoughts constantly switching back to his yard, he literally could not concentrate on anything else, especially not on thoughts such as "My lawn may not be the most important thing in the world." His mind kept jumping the track, so to speak, and returning to that one repeated concern.

To break Sam's preoccupation with the appearance of his yard, I found medication helpful, but not a complete cure. Medication is a temporary measure which in this case curbed and eased the unwanted, repetitive thoughts, such as "My yard must be absolutely perfect." Once that cycle of thinking was broken, I could guide Sam into other thoughts and behaviors. Behavior change achieves the same end that medication does; the drug gives the behavior change a chance to get started. As soon as Sam regained control, he didn't need the medicine anymore.

Sam still occasionally gets headaches, and once in a great while they stem from things like moles and rainy weather. He still loves puttering in his yard, but it is no longer an unavoidable obsession with him. He is a much happier, more contented man.

Easing the Stress

The specific advice I gave Mark and Joan, or the treatments used with Sam, helped them. But your headache triggers are uniquely your own. So I can only recommend in the most general terms how to find the triggers and minimize them as best you can. Don't be afraid to get creative.

Here are some other general ways to relieve stress.

Assertiveness training. "Oh, great," Joan grumbled. "Mark gets more assertive, and his headache goes away; but he gives everyone else a headache."

Actually, Mark didn't need assertiveness training. He already did well balancing the demands of others against his own needs. Some people, however, profit greatly from learning to more solidly express and meet their own needs in balanced and healthy ways.

Relaxation techniques. Some people think instantly of oriental or quasi-religious techniques such as yoga, but relaxation techniques are any methods that work for you.

A relaxation technique that is beneficial in helping many people overcome tension headaches simply involves going through the progressive muscle groups tensing the muscle very tightly then using that tension as a signal to relax. If you started with the biceps you would first breathe deeply then tighten your biceps. Feel the tension in your biceps and tell yourslef that this tension is the signal for you to relax. Respond to your signal to relax by exhaling and releasing the tension in your muscles. Eventually, once you feel tension anywhere, your body will recognize this signal and you will automatically begin to exhale and release the tension in your muscles. For thorough relaxation go through the following muscle groups tightening your muscles and then releasing the tension as you exhale: bicpes, neck, chest, back, gluteus maximus, thighs, and calves. By practicing this exercise you can learn to reduce the pain of tension headaches which are aggravated by neck muscle tension.

One of my patients keeps a tank of tropical fish just for relaxation. Says she, "I don't buy expensive fish. They are too hard to maintain. Besides, inexpensive kinds do the trick as nicely. Neon tetras are always a joy. I'll purchase at least half a dozen at a time so they can school together. Zebra danios like to school, also. Once in a while I'll introduce some hatchetfish. They skim along the top, looking comical—I love it! My neighbor keeps a tank of fancy playts. Beautiful fish!

"When I feel a headache coming on, I'll give the

kids crayons or a book or video, something to keep them occupied a while, and sit for a few minutes with a cup of tea and watch my fish. Just watch. So peaceful. It's sort of like a ritual."

Her comment *sort of like a ritual* means much. She has devised what is essentially a ritual for relaxing and calming her nerves. Can you devise a ritual for yourself, one that is uniquely your own, to achieve the same goal of relaxation?

Biofeedback. Biofeedback is a technique for which people are formally trained. Through it you regulate body and mental functions to reduce muscle tension and raise your skin temperature. The patients envision themselves in calm, safe, secure places. They imagine themselves at peace, without pain. The technique produces a pleasant, relaxed feeling.

Take a hot bath. A shower might work (and you ought to try it if you prefer a shower), but all those little pieces of water pummelling your body may not achieve the same relaxing effects as a quiet soak in warm water.

Rest and apply cold or heat to your head. The classic cartoon of the miserable headache sufferer with an icebag blobbed on his head is no joke. Some people find cold relaxes them; others prefer heat. Try both and see which works better for you.

Easing the Pain

"I'm sorry," Mark said, "but most of the time I can't do any of those relaxation things. I can't soak in a hot bath at work or stick an icebag on my head while I drive home—you see what I mean."

I certainly do. At this point we have to mute the

headache on one of the other sides of the triangle—
blood vessel control or nerve ending control. That requires drugs. Here's a rundown of various nonnar-
cotic analgesics. Some are specialty or prescription
drugs. None, with ordinary use, cause dependency.

Aspirin. Everybody knows aspirin. However, please
don't offer aspirin to children. In children it can trigger a life-threatening illness, Reye's Syndrome. Aspirin causes stomach upset, even ulcers, in some adults.
Coated aspirin may help those persons, but it works
more slowly.

Acetaminophen. This is the active ingredient in Tylenol. Acetaminophen is sold under other brands too.
Excedrin has acetaminophen plus caffeine. Be sure to
read labels!

Non-steroidal Anti-inflammatories (NSAID's). The
most common NSAID is ibuprofen, found in many over-
the-counter brands like Nuprin, Advil, and Motrin.

Other choices include Naproxen (Anaprox, Mapro-
syn), piroxicam (Feldene, touted as a 24-hour pain reliever; take it once a day), sulindac (Clinoril), tolmectin
(Tolectin), fenoprofen (Nalfon), indomethacin (Indocin), diclofenac (Voltaren), meclofenamate sodium
(Meclomen), Relafen, and Toradol. These prescription
remedies may cause significant side effects and, with
long-term use, may cause ulcers, and should always
be taken with food.

Narcotic drugs for extreme cases only, and then for
only limited use, include:

Morphine, Dilaudid, Codeine, Demerol, Numor-
phan, Dolophine Percodan, Vicadin, and Talwin.

If the headaches don't respond to mild analgesics,
try the ones recommended for migraine, starting with

low doses. You may want to ask your doctor about a low dosage of a tricyclic antidepressant such as Elavil for its pain inhibiting effects.

Rebound

Patty suffered frequent tension headaches. "Very well," she reasoned, "if a big dose of aspirin takes care of my headache" (she was taking three tablets initially, with two every three hours thereafter), "a small dose taken regularly should prevent them. Besides, aspirin is good for preventing heart problems, right?"

She also figured that since different over-the-counter analgesics contained different drugs that approached pain relief in different ways, taking two different drugs at once would double the pain-relieving effect. Before long she was suffering headaches daily and popping an amazing quantity of over-the-counter aids—ten Anacin tablets and twenty Tylenol tablets a day!

Patty did not think her daily headaches were all that out of the ordinary; her mother, too, suffered daily headaches. Rather, Patty saw a doctor because her husband forced her to.

"Her irritability, restlessness, and insomnia are driving me nuts," he fumed. "PMS is one thing, but this is ridiculous. Besides, she seems weak. I don't know how to explain it. She doesn't seem able to do as much as most other women can."

She admitted she was experiencing memory problems and difficulty concentrating. Her family doctor recognized depression as one of her symptoms.

Her doctor explained that the problem was rebound headache. It's also called medication induced or analgesic headache. Although she was not using any medication that itself causes addiction or dependency, she had in fact become psychologically dependent by adapting to her daily doses. These constant doses of pain reliever were causing neurochemical effects that were actually giving her a headache. In response she took still more analgesics. The cycle spiraled out of control. Remember the body as a chemical factory? She was messing up her body's natural chemistry by overloading it with other chemicals.

The first step in helping patients with recurring rebound headaches is to detoxify them. This usually involves a hospital stay, and the withdrawal symptoms are much like those caused by any other drug dependency. Patty required hospitalization. Her doctor used dihydroergotamine to ease her withdrawal. Once her body was cleansed of the trouble-making chemicals, she could take the second step. That was to work on her headaches with the same techniques Mark used. She learned to avoid or treat her headaches without resorting to excessive doses of medication.

A success story? Not this time. Within eight months, Patty was back to her old pattern of medication dependency, and the resulting symptoms—weakness, recurring headaches, irritability—were even more severe. Persons suffering rebound headache all too frequently relapse, as Patty did. Patty's underlying, unresolved emotional issues had to be addressed and treated before she could hope to see lasting relief from the rebound headaches. She saw no improvement until her husband, with emotional issues of his own, sought counsel as well.

Working Together

Patty and her husband, Joan and Mark—it often takes two to achieve improvement and eventual success.

Joan was doing some assertiveness repatterning of her own. She felt terrible that Mark's comfort depended so directly on her own health. "For crying out loud, Mark! When I'm down with a headache, let the house go. You don't have to vacuum and do the laundry just because it happens to be the day I usually do them. If you run out of underwear, go buy another package of it or something."

This was a huge step forward for Joan, a great revision in her own priorities and thinking. She came to grips with her own need to be perfect and learned to let go a little. Suddenly, she became impatient with Mark because he had not yet realized and acknowledged what she was learning.

Finally, therefore, let me counsel patience. When couples such as Mark and Joan work together on related problems, they will not march along together in perfect rhythm. They will leapfrog, one person seeing progress as the other lags, and then the lagging teammate forging ahead. Be patient with each other. Support each other. You'll arrive at the same end eventually—the alleviation of headaches as well as the deepening of important personal relationships.

"A migraine is not the worst headache you can get," claimed a man in my office named Warner. Joan would have argued the point vehemently, but Warner may be right. Very little, and perhaps nothing, equals the pain of the phenomenon called cluster headache.

The person suffering hangover would probably argue with both Joan and Warner. "Okay," the overindulger would say, "maybe a hangover doesn't equal your headaches for pure intensity, but for pure misery, there ain't nothing can come close!"

Let's look at these two kinds of headaches, first the cluster headache and then the hangover, which are unrelated except for one overriding similarity: they both cause unmitigated misery.

CHAPTER 8

Cluster Headaches

At exactly 3 P.M. each afternoon, the day shift lets out of the semiconductor plant as the evening shift comes on. Across town, a harsh buzzer announces the end of day at the junior high school.

At exactly 3 P.M. each afternoon, Warner Hansen, who teaches sciences at the junior high school, experiences the most severe, the most excruciating headache you can imagine. It's happened four days in a row. Each episode lasts about half an hour.

"So what?" you shrug. "If I had to teach science to a flock of eighth graders who don't care about learning it, I'd have a headache by three myself." But these are not tension headaches. They are not even migraines, exactly. We call them cluster headaches.

Cluster headaches are so called because they occur in groups, or clusters. They may strike as a swarm of many in a single day, or as a few each day over several days, or in some other periodic pattern. The sufferer may go for weeks or years between clusters before the next series of attacks occurs. During these periods of remission, he probably will experience no headaches whatever. One in ten victims of cluster headaches will suffer from chronic cluster, in which the attacks persist without remission—without a breather—for over a year.

How do you know if this is the problem you are suffering from?

Signs and Symptoms

Warner is typical in that most cluster sufferers are males between the ages of twenty and forty. Although his headaches occur during the afternoon, many sufferers are awakened in the night, often just after a period of REM (rapid eye movements) sleep.

Cluster headaches occur only on one side of the head, not both sides at once. Not switching sides, as migraine sometimes does. They stab, they burn intensely, but they do not pulsate. The victim tries in vain to lie still. He finds himself up and pacing about, even during the night.

Oke (his name is pronounced OH-keh) also suffers cluster headaches, and he would be first to agree with Warner that they are devastating, the worst pain known to man. Oke goes for a year or more without any problem whatever. Suddenly he gets five to ten fairly brief, slamming, stabbing headaches in a day. No warning. No culprit, such as wrong foods or behaviors. Not even national borders influence it. He's suffered them here in America, where he lives and works, and also in Sweden, where he visits family and friends frequently.

Oke's pain locates just under his right eye. His nose plugs up and runs, all congested. His right eye gets red and produces so many tears he can't see. Only the right eye, the one in front of the headache, looks this way. He breaks out in a sweat. His face turns red.

Oke's symptoms are typical. The excruciating bouts last from fifteen minutes to three hours. His headaches may just disappear for months, possibly even for years. Then it happens again without warning. Half of the sufferers report a stiff, achy neck, or shoulder pain.

As I mentioned, one in ten cluster sufferers becomes chronic. That is, the clusters occur with no remission, no headache-free period, for a minimum of one year.

Sometimes another type of headache will appear to be a cluster headache, as it did for Beth. "Look at this!" Beth said as she laid on my desk a page of neat columns. She had carefully tabulated, by date and severity, just about the same symptoms as are described for cluster headache. "But I'm not a man!"

She certainly wasn't. She was the wife of an acquaintance from church. And at first glance her problem indeed looked like cluster headaches.

She experienced attacks of severe, stabbing pain around her left eye. Usually, her attacks lasted half an hour or forty-five minutes. She'd get five or more such attacks a day over a period of days. "My nose runs, my eye really waters on that side, and the eyelid swells up. If that's not cluster, what is?"

It was chronic paroxysmal hemicrania (very much like cluster headaches), and it is primarily an adult woman's disease. We don't know any more about the mechanics of chronic paroxysmal hemicrania than we do that of cluster headaches. This doesn't mean that women don't have cluster headaches. Although most common in males ages twenty to forty, clusters can strike men or women of any age.

Causes

Unlike migraines, cluster headaches follow no significant genetic pattern; sufferers often report no family history of the problem. We believe that probable triggers include alcohol, certain foods, bright lights, and smoking. And yet, during those periods of headache-free remission, cluster sufferers can drink, eat, smoke, and suntan with impunity. The triggers get pulled only at certain, unpredictable times.

Many cluster patients smoke and drink a lot. A fourth of them have ulcer problems (about seven percent of the non-cluster population suffer ulcers). Most are high-powered, hard-driving, and perfectionistic. That describes Warner and Oke. That describes Beth too.

And yet, I've noticed, most cluster patients are passive in some areas of their lives, especially when it comes to taking care of themselves. For example, Warner's wife called the doctor, made an appointment for her husband, and literally picked him up after school and brought him in. She discussed the symptoms as Warner sat beside her, practically mute. When the doctor could not manage the headaches, she took Warner to another doctor. At no time did Warner undertake responsibility for his own cure.

Cluster headaches used to be called histamine headaches because doctors found that injections of histamine could trigger them in response to allergens causing itchy, red, teary eyes, weakness, and nasal congestion. Stress can precipitate histamine release, but no clear link exists between stress itself and cluster headaches.

Treatment

When you get a simple tension headache, you take your medicine; perhaps half an hour to an hour later the medicine takes hold, and you get on with your life. Cluster headaches attack so quickly and violently that the victim does not have the luxury of waiting half an hour for his medicine to grab. For that reason, doctors usually look for something that can prevent the episodes, defusing them before they happen. Clusters, however, are so thoroughly unpredictable that doctors usually have to resort to medication first, to take advantage of their preventative effects. But there are other ways to combat clusters besides pills!

One thing, which sometimes works, is simply to pay attention to your sleep-wake cycle. Everyone moves to a certain circadian rhythm, a daily pattern of behaviors. Some of us are morning folk who don't mind getting up so early we awaken the rooster. Others of us don't begin to function until ten A.M. Then along comes something like daylight saving time, or a change in your shift at work, and the circadian rhythms have to readjust.

Doctors have noted that a cluster series sometimes commences about ten days after the patient has abruptly shifted his daily rhythms. If you or someone you know suffer cluster headaches, it just might pay dividends to carefully monitor and control bedtimes and waking times. Keep to a set, nonviolable daily schedule as much as possible. When change is inevitable, such as a shift to daylight saving time, make it slowly, a little at a time, over an extended period, so that your daily rhythm is not jolted.

Obviously, in our clock-metered world, this isn't going to be possible very often. But if you abort a single cluster series before it occurs, it's worth it. The other alternative for aborting clusters before they occur is taking medication.

The best use of medication is on a daily basis, as preventative rather than abortive treatment. Many medications can help in preventing cluster headaches before they start. One option is verapamil (Calan, Isoptin). This can cause fatigue and complicate some heart problems, but overall it's quite safe.

If the patient is relatively young, less than thirty-five years old, we may start him on methysergide (Sansert). If that's not effective within a few weeks, we'll switch him to Prednisone, possibly in combination with verapamil. Methysergide has far fewer serious side effects than Prednisone does. Prednisone can cause problems in people with ulcers, heart or circulation problems, high blood pressure, and serious adrenal gland problems, so its use is best limited to a few weeks.

Lithium sometimes is effective for chronic cluster headaches as well as with the more common episodic cluster. Older men in particular seem to respond well to the drug. Patients on lithium must have frequent blood tests to be sure blood levels do not go up high enough to cause severe side effects or organ damage. Valproic acid, a medicine used to prevent seizures, can also help prevent clusters but, like lithium, it needs frequent blood tests and is consequently inconvenient.

Stopping a cluster series once it starts is much more difficult than preventing it. One very effective treatment for a cluster in progress is 100 percent oxygen. The oxygen tank and mask wait right at bedside. The moment the first sign of an attack occurs, the victim claps on the mask and inhales pure oxygen for ten minutes. If the oxygen is going to work at all it will work within ten minutes.

If you are a cluster headache sufferer, it may pay to rent the equipment and try it out. If it works, purchase your own rig. I have patients who own three separate oxygen delivery systems (a system consists of a refillable tank, a regulator to control the flow, and a clear plastic mask). One they stash at the bedside, one at the office desk, and one at the summer cabin.

Sometimes lidocaine, a local anesthetic, helps if it is dropped or sprayed into the nose on the affected side. It numbs certain nerve endings and that sometimes seems to ease the pain immediately.

About 80 percent of the time ergotamine will abort an attack, but you have to take it right away, almost before the attack begins to occur. You also have to absorb the drug into your system quickly. An aerosol that you can absorb through the lungs or a tablet placed under the tongue are the best methods. This is an excellent treatment for use after the headache starts.

Doctors are exploring the use of sumatriptan, the new migraine remedy, for handling cluster headaches. Sumatriptan comes in pre-loaded injectable doses that your doctor can teach you to use. It shows excellent promise.

Cafergot, the ergotamine plus caffeine compound, worked well for Warner because his attacks were somewhat predictable. Every day for about two hours before the expected attack—that is, about one o'clock in the afternoon—he took two tablets. The Cafergot headed off the attack. But Cafergot doesn't work well if that predictability is missing.

No response? Along comes DHE-45. You'll recall that dihydroergotamine is used for some migraine sufferers and is normally administered intravenously. Doctors are finding that it can quell clusters also, giving the prophylactic drugs, such as Sansert or lithium carbonate time to get started. The treatment requires several days at least of in-hospital care, as the DHE-45 is given every eight hours, but the relief makes it worth it.

Patients who simply do not respond to anything may have to consider surgery that cuts completely the nerves carrying the pain signals. These procedures are unpredictable and may actually worsen pain. They are truly a last resort.

"What about me?" Beth had been suffering her clusters of headaches for some time, and nothing over the counter worked. A pessimist at heart, she grumbled, "I'll probably end up being one of those resistant people."

I had good news for Beth. Chronic paroxysmal hemicrania responds beautifully to daily preventative doses of a drug called Indomethacin (Indocin). It would not have been appropriate for her if she had kidney problems or ulcers. Also, some other drugs interact poorly with indomethacin. Beth, however, was taking no other forms of medication. For her, it was an ideal cure.

What if she had some problem that precluded using the drug? In that case we would have first tried the other kinds of preventive therapies mentioned for cluster headaches. We would ask Beth to try inhaling 100 percent oxygen at the first sign of an attack or to use ergotamine in addition to the preventive medicine, if needed.

Other treatments are being tried and perfected as people come to appreciate better how devastating severe headaches can be. Cluster headaches used to be virtually unknown except to the people who suffered them. Doctors and patients alike are recognizing them more easily and coming to grips with them more effectively. But there is a headache that is completely preventable, known to virtually all by name if not by personal experience and laughed at more than just about any other malady you can think of.

The hangover.

Let us explore that next.

CHAPTER 9

The Hangover

Pete was a blaster on a western dam project. Usually, Pete would loudly and thoroughly warn everyone in the area about a pending detonation with this announcement over the public address system: "ATTENTION ALL UNITS! ATTENTION ALL UNITS! I'M GOING TO SHOOT!"

Beeeeeeep. The warning whistle would blare.

KA-BOOM!

One particular weekend, however, Pete partied much too hearty. Monday morning, he came to work with a head too big to fit in the Astrodome. In a soft, muffled voice he radioed, "Attention all units. Attention all units. I'm going to shoot as quietly as I possibly can."

Beep.

Poof.

The High Price of Indulgence

All manner of jokes and crude remarks await the poor soul who lets it be known he's suffering a hangover. Although a headache is not the sole symptom of hangover, it overshadows almost everything else that could go wrong with a person except perhaps the loss of a body part. Hangovers are in no way funny to those experiencing them.

Of course, the best way to avoid hangovers is to avoid alcohol altogether. One only has to read the grim statistics concerning alcoholism to realize it brings about monumemtal tragedy in countless lives. So, the best remedy is abstinence; but, we will deal with the medical aspects of alcohol use, including hangovers.

Just a few weeks ago, a truck driver friend of Pete's draped his arms over the tailgate of his pickup truck and shook his head as he popped his can of Pepsi. "Nope," Gary drawled. "No sir, I don't care what those migraine people claim about the worst headache imaginable. It's clear to me they never had a hangover or they wouldn't say that." The man knows whereof he speaks. He was an alcoholic for most of his adult life, intimately acquainted with the costs of overindulgence.

And everyone knows that overindulgence is indeed the culprit in the case of a hangover. However, hangovers are not the only headaches alcohol can generate, and the beverages we associate with alcohol are not the only places it is found. Alcohol sometimes occurs as an ingredient in products other than beverages, such as cough syrups, mouthwashes, and nearly all over-the-counter medicines. Whatever form the alcoholic substance takes, it will have two components: the alcohol itself (often a small percentage) and an assortment of *congeners*. Congeners are all the other chemicals, including water, in that particular beverage or other product, and they may have a profound effect on headaches.

The Chemistry of Alcoholic Substances

Jay, eager to appear sophisticated as well as manly, swills a couple of shots of vodka. His buddy Joe, however, is a small-town, good ol' boy with no interest at all in sophistication. He drinks a beer or two. Joe is certain that because he's drinking beer, he's getting a lot less alcohol than Jay. Shucks, everybody knows that. Jay, too, is certain he can handle his alcohol because everybody knows vodka does not produce a hangover.

Everybody knows. There is more folklore and misinformation about alcohol and its beverages than just about any other substance man consumes. Think about it: How much myth and pseudo-knowledge do you know that plumbs the mysteries of, say, broccoli? But alcohol is only one small part of the mélange of strange chemicals that make up a beverage. The congeners, which are all the other chemicals, produce their own effects independently. Sometimes they react in unpredictable ways with each other or with the alcohol, as well. The effects of alcohol are greatly complicated by the congeners, and the ways all that interacts inside you.

The Alcohol Itself

Jay and Joe listened to too many old wives' tales. "Everybody knows," indeed. They both had a lot of learning to do if they wanted to understand what actually went on as they drank. Their misconceptions, though, are common ones that many people share.

Dosage. The amount of alcohol different beverages contain, of course, varies widely. Beer has less, in that the percentage of alcohol is lower. Wine has a moderate percentage, and hard liquors—Jay's vodka, for example—carry the highest percentage of alcohol. However, Joe's beer represents a lot more volume than Jay's shot of vodka. Joe and Jay are both receiving about the same amount of alcohol per serving.

As a rough rule of thumb, then, a shot of hard liquor, a glass of wine, and a regular size beer (about twelve ounces) all deliver similar quantities of alcohol.

Effects. Alcohol is a vasodilator; it relaxes the fine muscles of blood vessels so that they expand. For some people, particularly people who are susceptible to vascular headaches such as migraine, the last thing you want is something dilating blood vessels rapidly. You'll remember that's what happens as a migraine begins. This is why a lot of migraineurs are teetotalers. They know alcohol can trigger a headache.

For a variety of reasons, alcohol should not be used in any form in conjunction with many medications. Because it dilates vessels, it can counteract important vasoconstrictors. It works synergistically with many drugs as well. That is to say, the effect of the drug and the alcohol together can be detrimental or even lethal, even though the presence of either one alone would ordinarily pose no problem. One of the effects of these unhappy synergistic responses is often headache.

Check with your doctor to find out if your medication can react with alcohol.

Because congeners contribute to hangover headache, you shouldn't mix beverages when you're drinking. You're ingesting an inordinate number of exotic chemicals with each kind of beverage, and these can interact unpredictably to cause headache. What a hodgepodge you're dumping in your system!

When we ask someone to itemize all the foods and beverages consumed, as I did with Mark, we ask for information on alcoholic beverages in detail. Mark does not drink, so he was avoiding all those chemicals. If he did drink, he would be asked to identify the beverages consumed by kind, variety, and quantity, and the time of day. Example:

Monday evening, 7/12, with dinner: 2 12-oz. cans light beer

Saturday evening, 7/24, before dinner: 1 shot whiskey

Tuesday, 8/2, with dinner: 1 4-oz. glass white wine

Taking a beverage with a meal does not alter the way the alcohol will be processed, but it will usually delay its effects. Also, it changes somewhat how the congeners are handled. You can see how complex this business is getting.

Because the chemical makeup of every person on earth is uniquely his or her own, every person will perceive the same chemicals differently. When Joe tastes a beer, he may not be experiencing the same sensations and flavors his buddy is. Similarly, his body chemistry may treat beer differently from his buddy's after it goes down. Even if the content of a particular beverage is consistent, its effects vary with different people.

Another important factor affecting dosage is plain old body weight. Also, research shows, in fact, that different races and tribes of human beings share a widely varying genetic ability to process alcohol. This means that some people may get alcohol headaches while others do not.

Two other obvious factors separate A and B, age and gender. Many people tend to have less tolerance for alcohol as they get older. That is, a dose that used to be processed comfortably now causes a hangover. And we're beginning to learn how markedly different are the general body chemistries of men and women. Each person has a different level of tolerance for alcohol.

Your response to alcoholic beverages then, both to the alcohol itself and to the congeners in them, will be uniquely your own. It cannot be accurately predicted by the nature of the beverage, your size, your age, your gender, your race, or any other factor. Your body chemistry may or may not tolerate alcohol or its congeners. The question you must answer that no one else can is "What effect does it have on me?"

Effects. "I never drink red wine," says May, a woman of about thirty. "Just a few ounces gives me a horrible headache within three hours or so. White wine? No problem. It's just certain reds. My minister, bless him, even changed his brand of communion wine for me."

Since millions of people enjoy red wines without repercussions, this problem sounds like it's May's alone. Not at all. Any person sensitive to histamines can have a problem with reds, and with certain other beverages as well. Most red wines, whose color derives from the grapeskins, contain considerable histamines.

Histamines are vasodilators. There's that word again. It tells you that migraineurs and sufferers of cluster headaches try to avoid red wines and other histamine-laden drinks. May, who does not ordinarily suffer migraines, happens to have a body chemistry that is strongly affected by that particular chemical.

Roy has an even more definitive quirk in his body chemistry: he cannot tolerate the alcohol itself. His body tells him instantly if he forgot to read the label of a medicine containing alcohol. For him, small amounts make a big impression.

He grimaced as he asked one day, "Why put alcohol in this stuff in the first place?"

Good question. There is a legitimate answer. Alcohol dissolves a number of chemicals that are insoluble in water. Alcohol itself, however, mixes easily with water (unlike oil, for instance). Therefore, to extract certain desired substances that are insoluble in water, you dissolve them in alcohol first. Then, in essence, you dissolve that tinctured alcohol in water. By that roundabout way, you bring the desired substances into water solution.

Vanilla extract has a high alcohol content because the alcohol is necessary to extract—that is, dissolve out—certain flavor chemicals. Water wouldn't do the trick. When you cook with the vanilla extract, most of the alcohol dissipates, for alcohol evaporates at a lower temperature than does water. But that doesn't help Roy. The poor guy has a real hard time with vanilla.

The chemicals in the beverage itself are only part of the problem. The body processes alcohol by breaking it down into other toxic chemicals, and these secondary chemicals go on to produce their own effects.

Just how does the body handle alcohol, and how does that in turn influence headaches?

Dealing with Hangover

"If I had a dollar for every hangover cure my so-called friends have inflicted on me over the years, I'd be able to buy Toledo." Gary can laugh about it now. But when he was in the throes of alcoholic overindulgence, he tried them all. A few of them nearly killed him. It helps to understand a few things about how your body processes alcohol.

Alcohol is not digested directly in the same way a slice of peanut-buttered bread, for example, is digested. The stomach handles the protein of the bread and the peanut butter, turning it into amino acids, which are absorbed into the blood for transport to cells. Meanwhile, the small intestine processes the carbohydrates. Again, the end products, sugars and acetic acid, go into the blood stream for transport to other parts of the body. In the small intestine, too, the fats are broken down by the action of bile that is dumped into the intestine from the liver. The broken down fats are then absorbed into the blood stream for final processing in the liver. Eventually, the nutrients of everything you eat end up in your blood.

Alcohol avoids all that lengthy middle-man processing by hopping straight into the blood stream and proceeding to the liver, brain, and all other body organs.

Alcohol, like sugar, can be absorbed through some membranes directly into the blood. As any drinker can tell you, you don't have to wait any length of time for it to affect you. As the amount of alcohol in your blood rises, it begins to cause the effects we lump together in the term *drunkenness*. The higher the alcohol level, the more pronounced the effects.

But the liver can only break down a certain amount of alcohol at a time. The liver's alcohol metabolism is slow and plodding and steady. It proceeds at its own pace. The alcohol not yet broken down simply continues circulating through the body, carried in the blood, until the liver gets around to it.

There is, in short, no way to speed up or slow down the liver's work in breaking alcohol down into other chemicals for elimination by the kidneys. (The alcohol eventually ends up as sugars which, if not burned, are turned into fat—the infamous beer belly.) A person with a high blood alcohol content cannot reduce it quickly by some magical means. There is no sobering-up cure to speed the process.

"That's probably just as well." Since drying out, Gary has been reading up on the chemistry of alcoholism. "With all the break-down products the liver makes out of alcohol, you wouldn't want that stuff dumped on you quickly." He's right. The body can handle the waste products and break-down chemicals of alcohol metabolism if it receives them in slow, measured quantities.

. . . To a point. And here's where the hangover, excuse the expression, raises its ugly head.

The hangover headache results from the by-products created as the liver processes blood alcohol. Since the processing takes a while, the hangover usually occurs several hours later—the morning after. Even more poisonous and debilitating are the congeners, and the products and by-products that come from processing them. As a general rule, alcoholic drinks with the hairiest assortments of complex congeners produce the hairiest headaches. This is why the myth arose that vodka does not generate a hangover. It does, but because its congeners are fewer and simpler, its aftermath is not as excruciating.

You can do a few things to prevent making a bad thing worse. Avoid loud noise if possible, including shouting and blaring music. Be thankful you aren't Pete the blaster, whose business is loud noise. If you are a smoker, smoking a cigarette may soothe your nerves, but the nicotine may make the headache worse. Too, although alcohol is a drink, it is a diuretic (which stimulates the body to excrete fluids), causing dehydration which exacerbates the headache pain. Drinking liquids can help you past that.

You can also do a few things to mitigate the discomfort a little. Rest. That's probably the biggest help. Caffeine is a vasoconstrictor, so strong coffee and tea might help. Coffee, however strong, will *not* sober a person up. It cannot speed up the process of removing alcohol from the blood. It will, however, help the blood vessels close back down.

Aspirin can actually make headache pain worse, and is best avoided in cases of hangover headache. Vitamins are important for nutrition, especially if your diet is not well balanced. (They are not useful, however, in treating hangover headache.)

Alcohol is not the only cause of hangovers. Other drugs and substances, most of them legal and even beneficial, can cause severe headaches. Let us look at them next.

CHAPTER 10

Toxic Stuff

It's a brand new building, state of the art, gorgeous in the details of its interior decoration. Forty-seven percent of the office staff who work inside it report almost daily headaches and other symptoms.

Pete the blaster, whose hangover we talked about in chapter nine, is the only guy on the construction project who gets frequent headaches. It can't be alcohol; he's given up drink.

Marjorie just returned from Australia, where she worked for two years on a missions outreach. She's come to accept her relentless daily headaches as an unfortunate fact of life, like monsoons, tropical diseases, and cab drivers who charge too much.

All these people are suffering needlessly.

Headache is one of the most common symptoms generated by toxins. You've often heard the term *substance abuse* in its usual meaning: misuse of or addiction to controlled substances such as marijuana and illicit drugs. But its full meaning covers a much, much wider scope of substances, including licit drugs, and the abuse may not be voluntary.

We medical practitioners use another related term when talking about toxic substances, *acute use*. Acute use is a very large dose that is received by the body all at once. For example, Pete's hangover was caused by an acute use of a potentially toxic substance, alcohol.

Toxins occur everywhere. The high-minded but misguided person who would make the world safe from toxic substances lives in a fool's paradise. We talked about the toxins in coffee back in chapter five. You'll recall that many plants—most, in fact—contain toxins and other chemicals to discourage browsers. We mentioned also that many plants' toxic defense chemicals can react in susceptible people. But they are not the only ingestible headache-producers to watch out for.

We could classify headache-generating toxins two ways: those which do their nefarious work from within our bodies, called *endotoxins*, and those that come in from outside, called *exotoxins*.

Toxins Within

Most body malfunctions can produce headaches. Any little disorder can be a big culprit. In this case the headaches are a side issue; the important item is the malfunction itself. The sooner you discover and deal with organic dysfunctions, the better your general health will remain. The kidneys filter out hundreds of poisonous toxins, and any kidney problem can quickly cause a build-up of toxins that can cause headache.

Also, many viral and bacterial infections, for example, frequently cause headache because of the toxins they produce.

Calcium imbalance can also cause headaches. When we mention calcium, most patients think of little old ladies losing calcium in their bones to osteoporosis. That is indeed a problem. But men and women both need an optimum calcium level for their nerves to function properly. Too little, and nerves don't transmit their signals well. Excessive calcium intake is just as bad and can also cause severe headaches.

Our friend Marjorie, the missionary back from Australia, had another problem, a rickettsial infection she picked up from a tick bite. Because she had remained virtually disease free during most of her two-year stay, and because the fever that accompanies this infection was so minimal as to be almost unnoticeable, she didn't think about the tick bite. She attributed her headaches to the drastic time change and the culture shock of returning stateside.

I mention Marjorie to illustrate an important point for you to remember. While the vast majority of infections are garden variety bacteria and viruses, there are a lot of other infections that can cause headaches. Spotted Fever, for instance, is uncommon so when it does occur, it can easily be missed. See your doctor if you feel ill in any way along with your headache.

When assaying possible causes for your headaches, particularly dull, heavy, recurring ones, don't neglect the possibility of infection. These questions might help:

1. In the last few weeks, have I been around people with noticeable infections (including people recovering from them)?
2. Have I been traveling to or through exotic places where I might have picked up some bug I'm not

used to? *Exotic* here means overseas, of course, but it also means Louisiana if you lived in Maine all your life, or Maine if you grew up in Louisiana ... habitats which differ widely from what you're used to and therefore will harbor germs you're not used to.

3. Have I visited places where people seem to get sick a lot (a particular workplace or situation)?

4. Might I have been exposed to infection by a visitor who came to see me, or by others in a common area (being sneezed upon at the mall, that sort of thing)?

5. What have my kids brought home from school lately? Kids are a smorgasbord of infectious organisms during the school year.

Treating these infections is treating the headaches that come from these sources. Most likely, over-the-counter pain remedies that you would use for tension headaches will work here as well, providing temporary relief until the infections themselves are brought under control.

Toxins from Without

Barbara got a touch of stomach flu, accompanied by a headache, and she has no idea from whom she caught it. When a friend suggested food poisoning, she said, "No, I didn't eat anything my husband didn't eat also, and he's fine. Couldn't be that."

Improperly Handled Foods

What Barbara said was true, but she forgot that on Monday she ate leftover chicken from Sunday afternoon, which had been sitting on the kitchen counter for quite a while. Her husband indeed ate the same chicken she did, but not on Monday. Many health officials claim that a lot of what is dismissed as stomach flu is actually food poisoning from improperly prepared or stored foods.

Improperly handled foods therefore rank as an important cause of headaches and attendant illness. People with food poisoning are going to feel rotten regardless what they do or take. It's one of those things that just has to run its course, and usually stops by itself in 1–3 days.

Food Additives

Chemicals added to food rank high as headache producers in people who are susceptible to them, and many people are. Monosodium glutamate (MSG) is probably the most familiar culprit. Some call this headache Chinese Restaurant Syndrome because oriental restaurants so often use MSG as a flavor enhancer. The headache feels like one of those tension headaches, with a throbbing band of pain and pressure in your temples and forehead. Besides the headache, you feel pain in your chest and a hot flush all over your upper body. Your face seems tight or under pressure.

Dyes also affect some people. So do nitrates and nitrites, substances that migraineurs and other headache sufferers quickly learn to avoid. Avoidance is the best cure for such headaches too.

Excessive Vitamins

Vitamins? Unfortunately, you can get too much of a good thing. People who take excessive amounts of certain vitamins, mostly vitamins A and D and niacin, can get bad headaches (we're talking thousands of units daily here). Other symptoms go along with it. Vitamin D overdose leads to gastrointestinal distress as well as headache. Excess vitamin A causes a strange thickening and hardening of the skin and cracks and sores in the mouth area. Nicotinic acid, or niacin, is a vasodilator, and therefore should be avoided by migraineurs. People who want to stay away from vasodilators might ask about a niacin substitute, niacinamide.

Minerals

Exposure to minerals can be a source of headache pain.

Copper intoxication usually happens through the water supply. Consider it a possibility if you have copper plumbing or your water is delivered through copper pipelines. Symptoms other than headache include nausea, diarrhea, excessive secretion of saliva, and a metallic taste. At least one researcher suggests that migraineurs ought to avoid copper intake.

Lead is a familiar poison, thanks to an intensive public education program about the health dangers of lead. Lead-free paints are replacing the older paints that literally bring the poison into your home. Unleaded gasoline is further reducing environmental lead levels. I mention it here because children who don't necessarily manifest other symptoms of lead poisoning may have headaches from it.

While we're discussing lead, don't forget the other additives in today's gasolines. If you work around petroleum products, keep them in mind as a possible source.

Manganese is another headache-producing mineral.

"I've just been working on Groote Eylandt. I bet you don't know where Groote Eylandt is," boomed a grinning Aussie. From him, though, it sounded, like Oy bet you down't now where Growdy Oylant is.

The Aussie was a manganese miner just returned to civilization for medical treatment. He was developing Parkinson's disease, it appeared—severely impaired nerve function and motor control. His intense headaches, poor appetite, and general blahs didn't help.

The miner inhaled enough manganese, his doctors determined, that it upset his enzyme complexes. Once he got out of the mines, he did much better. Manganese is not mined much in this country (we import almost all of our manganese), but it is used widely in industry. It goes into batteries, the strongest steel and bronze, and some other products, such as paint and industrial chemicals. If you work with manganese in factories, be aware of the possibilities of manganese as a cause of vicious headaches.

Pesticides can make you ill. Be extremely careful in how you use them and in your children's exposure to them. If you suspect your headache is due to a pesticide, call your doctor or a poison control center for advice.

Pollution, carbon monoxide (CO). It is a clever coincidence that Tolkien's Hobbits battled a fire-and-smoke-breathing dragon named Smaug. The millions of people worldwide who suffer during conditions of heavy smog would insist that smog is as dangerous and destructive a dragon as Smaug. Unfortunately in today's world, pollution severe enough to cause illness is easy to find.

The health enthusiast who runs in smoggy weather or in heavy traffic may well fall victim to a pollution-induced or CO-induced headache. Auto exhausts are not the only source of carbon monoxide, however. Any fire that does not burn its fuel completely may be producing CO. Keep a wary eye out for it when using a charcoal grill, certain open-flame kerosene space heaters, or open fires, such as a campfire in a partially enclosed shelter. A headache is a big red flag telling you to get out of there immediately.

Your blood carries oxygen around through your body by picking it up on the red blood cells passing through your lungs. Carbon monoxide poisons you by attaching to your red blood cells before oxygen can do so. Because it attaches more easily than does oxygen, it literally shoulders out the oxygen. So firmly does it stick to the receptor area where the oxygen ought to be, the red blood cells have an almost impossible time getting rid of it. There it stays, merrily riding around and around through your body, keeping oxygen from attaching to the cells, offering no help at all to your oxygen-starved cells. You remain oxygen-starved, therefore, even when you're breathing good air again.

In addition to headache, symptoms of carbon monoxide poisoning include feeling faint and nauseated. Dilated pupils are a sign. If the person who has breathed carbon monoxide shows patches of redness on the face or chest, get medical help immediately. That person needs the additional oxygen and the detoxification a hospital can provide.

Workplace hazards might be considered specialized cases of pollution for the most part. The office workers I mentioned at the beginning of the chapter were suffering from the pollution inside what we call "a sick building." However the polluting chemicals are introduced—through the newly installed carpet, through the air conditioning system, by some mechanism that cannot be determined—a number of people may be sensitive to the introduced molecules. Headaches are sometimes the first sign of trouble.

The solution, other than taking the usual analgesics for symptomatic relief, must lie with the building owner or manager; over that person, unfortunately, the employee has little control. The wise owner or manager will take whatever steps are necessary to remedy the problem immediately. The headaches alone are costing big bucks in reduced employee efficiency and productivity, and absenteeism escalates in sick buildings.

"Hmph," snorted a friend of our family. "I remember when buildings were plastered or paneled with wood inside. Gets hot? You open a window. Too cold? Close it. No fancy climate control. Just fresh air."

However much he might yearn for the good old days (if there ever was such a thing), the present reality is that we are inundated by strange and unusual chemicals at work, at home, and at play. Building interiors are not made of plain wood and plaster these days. Windows that you can open mess up the climate control system. Considering how many substances we live and work with compared to how many our parents knew, not all that many cause problems. Tackle the problem by trying to find the source, and ameliorate the headache pain with analgesics in the meantime.

Pete, the blaster, faces a workplace problem of another sort. Why is he plagued by recurrent headaches when no one else on the site is? A question like that usually can be answered by looking for whatever it is that the headache sufferer is uniquely exposed to. In Pete's case it was the explosives. He was sensitive to certain chemicals he absorbed while working closely with them.

Pete saw as his choices: putting up with it, going into some other line of work, or protecting himself differently. He chose the latter. Now he sets his charges wearing a hazmat suit. He looks a little silly (his friends call him Moonwalker now, and he gets all sorts of gibes about "Shooting me to the moon"), but he no longer suffers blaster's headache.

Any workplace situation has the potential to be a headache source (here's your cue to get a few jabs in about the boss). These sources can come from unexpected quarters. Welders, for example, can get the "zinc shakes" from inhaling vaporized, oxidized zinc while welding galvanized (zinc coated) steel. If headaches are a problem for you, turn detective. Ask questions, particularly about the chemistry of various processes with which you make contact. Most important, be certain to report the incidence of headaches, nausea, or other symptoms to building authorities. The powers that be can't fix a condition they don't know exists, and they are required by law to keep track of health problems.

Prescription and nonprescription drugs. To control her migraines, Joan took 2 milligrams of ergotamine orally daily for three months. The migraines are avoided, but now she suffers a headache generated by the ergotamine itself. It's not localized like migraines are; it pulsates somewhat, and it just hangs on forever. When she goes off the ergotamine she will get an ergotamine-withdrawal headache. If she goes off the ergotamine, the migraines will probably return. Life is not fair.

Actually, it is. We put her on sumatriptan and she's doing just fine. No headache.

Joan illustrates an excellent point. Drugs, even drugs given to alleviate headaches, can cause headaches. Both prescription and nonprescription drugs can be culprits. When checking with your doctor about the possibility that a certain drug may be giving you headaches, remember that three things are involved: the nature and identity of the drug itself (in Joan's case, ergotamine), the dosage (at a dosage less than 2 milligrams daily, Joan might have avoided the ergotamine headache, but the migraines might have returned), and the length of time the drug is used. Joan didn't start running into trouble until three months after she began the regimen. And don't despair. If adjusting dosage doesn't help you, there is often an alternative to be found that will work almost as well as the drug you are using.

In the box below, I've listed other drugs known to cause headaches. If you are routinely taking any of these, and nagging, recurrent headaches are a problem, discuss with your doctor the possibility of trying something else, at least for a while, as an experiment. Keep in mind that withdrawal may also pose a problem, as Joan discovered with her ergotamine.

For the longest time, Joan was unaware that her birth control pills were intensifying her migraines. They certainly were not the root cause of her headaches; she experienced migraine whether she remained on the pill or not. But we frequently find that in women who are already migraineurs, the pill can cause increased frequency and/or increased intensity in migraines. A British study found that one-third of women who went on the pill subsequently suffered migraines for the first time, although switching pills sometimes alleviates headaches.

Drugs That Can Cause Headaches

Caffeine	Nitroglycerine
Ergotamine	Ranitidine (Zantac)
Alcohol	Certain steroids
Birth control pills	Certain NSAIDs
Histamines	Hydralazine (a blood
Some antihistamines	pressure medicine)

One other drug deserves mention here. It is one of the very few drugs that many, many people shoot up with daily for no reason at all, and they do it legally: caffeine. Coffee is the most frequent source. A cup of regular coffee gives you 100 milligrams; a cup of decaffeinated about 3. A can of cola provides around 50. One American in five consumes more than 500 milligrams of caffeine daily.

Coffee is not the only source of caffeine, nor is it, at times, the only important one. Caffeine is also compounded as an ingredient in many over-the-counter drugs, such as Midol, Emperin, Bromo-Seltzer, Anacin, Excedrin, and a host of others. Read the label!

In excess of 200 mg per day, caffeine gives you a dull, thudding headache. It also makes you feel nervous, even shaky, and irritable, and can interfere with sleep.

Withdrawal from drugs. Mark, you may recall, suffered his own withdrawal headache when he went cold turkey off caffeine. Caffeine withdrawal is wicked. The headache is bad enough. But you also feel cranky and sleepy. You don't want to stir, let alone work or act alert. Pain relievers won't touch the headache. The withdrawal symptoms will occur about a day after you cut off the caffeine intake and may last several long, long days.

Although regular pain relievers won't touch the withdrawal headache, there is a cure. It's some hair from the dog that bit you: that is, to alleviate the caffeine-withdrawal headache, take just a little caffeine. One cup of coffee will do it. But you need about 100 milligrams (at least a cup of coffee) for the caffeine cure to work. One can of cola won't do it, in other words. You'll need two.

You can avoid the headache and all the nastiness if you taper off the caffeine gradually instead of stopping suddenly as Mark did. Calculate about how much you consume daily and deliberately ingest a little less each day over a period of, say, a week or two. Once weaned, perhaps you can take in small amounts of caffeine with no problem.

If you drink a lot of caffeine at work, either as coffee, tea, or colas, you might find yourself with a zinger of a headache on your day off unless you continue at least some caffeine intake. Many people who think they are getting weekend migraines are actually going into caffeine withdrawal. The bottomless coffee pot at work gives way to a hasty departure for the weekend destination, or getting an early start on the yard work, or going downtown to get the shopping done, or lubing the pickup truck, or whatever. Monitor your caffeine intake carefully in order to avoid both overuse and unintended withdrawal.

Other drugs can cause headaches upon withdrawal. Chief among them are the narcotics. Movies are made about people trying to quit such drugs. There are substances, Clonidine, for one, that can help ease the devastating symptoms during the withdrawal period.

There are seasons of the year when people are much more likely to take both prescription and over-the-counter remedies. Colds seem more prevalent in winter, for example. But the big onslaught against sensitive sufferers comes in spring and summer when the pollen blows. Allergies and seasonal irritations cause headaches as well as the familiar sneezing and the draining sinuses.

Let's look specifically at allergies.

CHAPTER 11

Oh, My Stuffy Sinuses!

If you think I'm allergic to something, you've got holes in your head!" Calling Stanley opinionated was putting it mildly.

"Yes. Exactly." Stanley's doctor smiled benignly.

Stanley, his arms crossed tightly across his chest, smirked at him. "Exactly what? That you have holes in your head?"

"I do. And so do you." So does everybody. And Stanley's holes in his head were giving him fits.

Stanley's wife brought him to the doctor because Stanley suffered what was essentially one long, continuous headache from April through August. He became more cantankerous than usual then and felt so miserable that he tended to make everyone else miserable. She claimed he was cantankerous enough the other seven months. She didn't need this as well.

Stanley was only forty-five, but he was prematurely gray and somewhat rotund, so he delighted in playing the part of the cranky old man. Not only did he crab and fuss, he was certain all his opinions were right. One of his opinions was that *allergy* was a term used by shiftless persons who want to avoid honest work and are too healthy to take sick leave legitimately. You never heard about allergies a hundred years ago, did you? And there were more diseases then. Allergies, Stanley pointed out, are a figment of the imagination.

Stanley was suffering a severe figment of his imagination. Said his doctor, "Humor me a little. Let's run a few tests to find any major irritants in your life."

Stanley gestured at his wife, apparently identifying one of his major irritants. But he put up with a series of patch tests and seemed to delight in the fact that they provide plenty of grist for complaint.

Stanley was allergic to Bermuda grass, certain weed pollens, and feathers. "Nonsense!" barked Stanley gruffly.

"It figures," his wife mused. "About April is when he starts cutting the grass frequently, and our lawn is Bermuda. And all summer he fiddles around with his homing pigeons."

"Doesn't he mow the lawn in September and October?" the doctor asked.

"No. That's when our nephew takes care of the house and pigeons and we go up to our cabin in Colorado." A light dawned in the wife's eyes. "And that's when the headaches taper off!"

Allergies

Headaches caused by allergy and other sinus problems may have a variety of sources. The allergens—that is, the agents to which you, or Stanley, react—are one source. Another is the effect on blood vessels that the allergic reaction may have. And the third source is the medications used to combat the allergy.

Stanley made some major changes in his surroundings. He built modifications in his pigeon cotes that limited his exposure to pigeon feathers and mites. He had a local boy come in and do the lawn during the day while he was at work. Certain that weed pollens in the air are also a figment of someone's imagination, he refused to get with a program of filtering them out. No matter. With two of his three major irritants reduced he improved so much he started avoiding summer weed pollens on his own. He didn't tell anyone, of course.

Is It a Sinus Headache?

Questions to Ask:

1. Does it wax and wane with a season or seasons?
2. Do other people suffer similarly at the same time you do? Have they identified a specific source or sources of irritation that you might explore?
3. Do these symptoms accompany your headaches:
    A. Rhinitis (runny or infected nose)
    B. Itching, irritated eyes
    C. Sneezing; tickling sensation in nose or throat
    D. Irritability, mood swings, memory lapses, dizziness, depression, anxiety
    E. Fatigue
    F. Aches and pains you don't normally experience
    G. Constipation or diarrhea
    H. Heart abnormalities
    I. Nausea
    J. Vaginal burning

Stanley illustrates an important point about allergies; most people are not neatly limited to a single irritant. Stanley, like most sensitive people, reacted to several unrelated agents. In fact, sensitivity to one agent usually implies sensitivity to others as well. This throws a clinker into any effort to find the allergy source by simple observation.

"If I stay away from Bermuda grass, and I feel better, then that must be an irritant." You probably won't be able to say that because although you manage to stay away from Bermuda grass, other irritants are masking the good effects. Until you have some idea what most of your irritants are, you can't cut out enough at once to see the difference. This is where professional testing comes in.

What about you? Do you get seasonal headaches? If so, during what season? Prime pollen sources vary with different parts of the country, as do their main season. For instance, in parts of the west in spring, the evergreens release enough pollen to literally turn parked cars chartreuse. Over most of the country, ragweed is a notorious irritant. Don't neglect weird possibilities; analyses in a few areas show marijuana as a major pollen source.

Major irritants—that is, agents that cause allergic reactions in large numbers of people—have long been identified as "the first place to look." They include various pollens (release of pollens occurs only during that plant's season of bloom; the plant is nonirritating when not in bloom); dust and the microscopic mites so often associated with dust, especially house dust; feathers; animal hair and dander (the dead skin flakes all mammals shed). Some people react allergically to some foods, particularly wheat, chocolate, and cow's milk products. Ask around about common allergy irritants in your area.

Incidentally, although allergic reactions are commonly called "hay fever," hay is rarely the culprit. More often it's the mold growing in the hay.

Also, at about the same time the headaches occur, does your nose get stuffy? Do your eyes start watering for no real reason? If so, it's time to investigate the possibility that your headaches are in fact allergy related. But Stanley, complex as his allergic reactions were, actually had a simple case with fairly simple solutions. Many people with a runny nose and headache suffer not just from allergies but from a plethora of problems that know no season. However, in the end, we believe that the stuffy nose is part of the culprit in sinus headaches.

Other Sinus Problems

As Stanley's doctor said, we all have holes in our heads—the hollow spaces behind our eyes, nose, and cheeks that keep the skull weight down. The spaces' location is such that a very thin partition separates the sinuses from the inside of our nose and the gums above the upper teeth. Anything that affects the nose usually also affects the sinuses.

Not only do the sinuses and nose lie so close together they affect each other, the sinuses have drainage channels that run into the nose. Infection from the nose can back up into the sinuses. If the sinuses become infected and clogged up, pressure develops and a headache may result. The by-products of the infection can cause headaches as well.

The indiscriminate daily use of nasal decongestants can actually contribute to a headache. After about four days they may not even affect the congestion anymore and can "backfire" to cause headaches.

The best known symptoms of allergic reactions in addition to headache are rhinitis (runny nose); red, itchy, watery eyes; sneezing; and perhaps irritability. Heaven knows, Stanley was irritable. But other possible symptoms that you don't immediately associate with allergy are fatigue, aches and pains, constipation or diarrhea, heart abnormalities, nausea, and vaginal burning. Other symptoms occasionally caused by allergies include memory lapses, dizziness, and depression. Sometimes anxiety and mood swings erupt.

These allergies contribute to sinus headaches, but we need to be sure they are actually causing the headaches before treating them.

We approach the treatment of sinus headaches as we approach other treatments; start with the simplest, easiest, and cheapest, and work up as necessary. (In this case, if standard sinus remedies don't do anything, you may not have a sinus headache after all. It is then time to start looking in other directions.)

Treating Sinus Headaches

The simplest treatment is not always the simplest. Avoiding the irritants. It is simplest—and therefore superior—because no medications are involved. But avoiding some agents can be far from simple. How do you avoid wheat or milk or eggs when so many things contain wheat? Airborne particles of dust, pollen, and animal dander are everywhere; there's no getting away from them. Another serious problem with avoiding irritants is knowing which irritants to avoid. You cannot always unmask all the culprits. Medical testing is essential here.

Tests by a doctor or an allergy clinic can tell you what irritates you and how badly. You may boil over like Job when a powerful allergen enters the room. You may show only a mild reaction to certain agents. Be advised before you walk in to the tests that they may not be conclusive. The tests are somewhat subjective, and results are not clear-cut.

Doctors may also sift out various sources of your problem by trying different drugs. Your reaction to those drugs tells the doctors what they are dealing with. Nasalcrom, a spray that blocks the release of histamine, may block the effects of allergic rhinitis and its attendant headaches.

Another product, Nasalide, is a steroid. It helps reduce swelling of nasal passages that can block sinus drainage. If it works well, you can probably be on steroid nasal sprays for the long term.

Over-the-Counter Relief

I could list all the over-the-counter remedies, but you can get the same list from the shelf at your pharmacy, and you're going to end up there anyway. Look for:

Antihistamines. These drugs keep the body from reacting too wildly to incoming irritants and other allergens.

Decongestants. The congestion that decongestants decongest, of course, is the clogging and dripping in your nose and sinuses (and sometimes extending into the eustachian tubes which lead from your throat into your ears). Your objective is to drain the sinuses, relieving the pressure and ridding them of the by-products of infection. Try milder dosages, and if they don't do much for you, beef the dosage.

Be advised that some drugs, both prescription and over-the-counter cause vasodilation to the extent that they actually produce headaches in susceptible people.

Nonprescription nonsteroidal decongestants often do the trick if the problem is nothing more than seasonal allergic irritation. If they do not, your second wave of attack is prescription drugs.

Sinus remedies can be delivered by various means, but the commonest is a nasal spray or an inhaler. The sensitive membranes of your nose and lungs pick up chemicals instantly and transmit them immediately to the blood stream. Too, inhalers deposit the medicine directly on the site.

When you're looking at inhalers, choose a system that prevents, to phrase the term delicately, backdraft. This is especially important when children or young adults are involved. An example of a delivery system I consider inadequate for kids or careless adults, is the bottle with a pointed delivery tip that you stick up into your nose. You squeeze the plastic bottle and deliver the medicine to your nasal linings. But if you relax your squeeze before the bottle is clear of your nose, you could drag some of the contaminants back into the bottle. There they sit inside the medicine, to be shot back into your nose with the next dose. Bacterial growth and infection result.

Sinus Headache Prongs of Attack

	Relief Achieved	No Relief Achieved
1. Determine if allergens or irritants are involved		
Nasalcrom	Allergies are a factor	Allergies are not a factor
Nasalide	Irritants are a factor	Irritants are not a factor
2. Avoid identified allergens and irritants. Avoid suspect foods . . . situations	†	Try over-the-counter remedies: • Antihistamines • Decongestants, such as non-prescription nonsteroidal decongestants
3. Over-the-Counter	†	Try prescription drugs
4. Prescription Drugs	†	Last resort: surgery on sinus linings

†Clinically conducted allergy tests

Sinus Problems That Resist Treatment

An alternative some people choose when all else fails is to have a surgeon cut back the linings.

"I reamed 'em out, and it didn't do much good," claims one.

"Best thing I ever did," claims another.

I don't personally recommend surgery for most people. In fact, it should be the last resort. There are usually better alternatives.

Persistent sinus problems—that is, the difficulties that simply do not respond to any effort you make—could suggest some deeper problem, and you should be sure to see a physician.

After you think you have nailed down what appear to be the causes of your headaches—everything from allergies and infections to stress and tensions at work—there remain a host of strange little sources that bother enough people frequently enough to be considered here. And an odd lot they are, as we shall see in the next chapter.

CHAPTER 12

Headaches from Other Sources

Frankly, this is embarrassing. This is really embarrassing," Gene admitted. His cheeks and neck flushed. "You've heard the line, 'Not tonight, dear. I have a headache.' Well, I get the headache *after* we make love."

His wife nodded agreement. "I feel so sorry for Gene, that he gets these headaches. That's bad enough. But he tends to, well, lose interest sometimes because of it. And it seems so weird, you know?"

"Sex" Headaches

Actually, sex headaches aren't all that weird; in fact, although they are uncommon, they are certainly not unheard of. They occur in both men and women, usually at about the onset of the most intense sexual excitement. We're not exactly sure what causes sex headaches.

Usually a sex headache is what we like to call an individual anomaly, just some little quirk in a person's physical makeup. Occasionally, though, it is a symptom of hypertension. You'll recall that high blood pressure does not normally produce a headache unless it gets really high. When a person with silent high blood pressure engages in intercourse, the activity and excitement can boost blood pressure, and headache pain results. That's why persons experiencing sex headaches should get a blood pressure check if they've not done so already.

In fact, knowing your baseline blood pressure is an excellent idea even if you don't get sex headaches. In the event of an illness or accident, the first thing medical caregivers want to know—and it is a most useful thing to them—is what your blood pressure is normally. With that information they can evaluate whether your blood pressure is stable, dangerously low, or dangerously high. So get your blood pressure checked anyway, and make sure you know what it is.

Some people get headaches when they engage in any exercise strenuous enough to cause the face to flush. Doctors believe that as hard physical exercise raises the sufferer's blood pressure and pulse rate, the smaller vessels do not dilate in time to literally take the pressure off the larger ones. The larger arteries stretch, and headache results.

Body Parts out of Alignment

"My dumb car is a squirrel!" a friend recently complained. "It's all over the road, especially on tight turns. Any little jiggle in the road surface, and it bucks like a bull. I try to take that lefthand curve as you're crossing railroad tracks down by Bakers', and it jumps into the oncoming lane! That's not healthy."

"Get the front end aligned," another friend advised.

"Oh, come on. A fraction of an inch in the front wheels can't make all that much difference."

But it did. She gave the wayward front end new shocks and a professional alignment. Now the car handles just fine, even down by Bakers'. A small misalignment in the human body can wreak just as much havoc, including headaches.

With ideal posture in human beings, the face is exactly vertical, the eyes level upon the world, the head upright. But the head and its face top off an extremely flexible skeleton that can very easily develop an off-center slant. That tilt must be corrected at or below neck level and usually the corrective influence is increased muscle tension on the "long" side. Persons with one leg noticeably shorter than the other may suffer headaches because of that asymmetry. When a person stands and walks, the hips should ride level, or nearly so. Anything which tilts the hips to one side or the other forces the muscles to counterbalance the tilt. Those reactions can lead to tension headaches and related problems.

In some persons, the bones forming one side of the pelvis are smaller than those forming the other. Small hemipelvis, it's called (*hemi* means half). The person walks, stands, and sits, literally at a slight slant. The upper body adjusts for the misalignment by curving slightly. The constant muscle action needed to keep the corrective curve in place causes tension.

Remember the two women discussing the relationship between tight muscles and tension headaches during snow driving? This adjustment has the same effect.

Scoliosis is curvature of the spine. It can be caused by the small hemipelvis just described or by misalignments in the spine itself. Whether it leads to headache or not, it should be attended to promptly. Scoliosis never just goes away, but can be reversed easily if treated in childhood.

Really poor posture, with no physical misalignment or deformity involved, can lead to headaches all by itself. Again, muscles constantly having to keep the head straight get tight and tense. The cure for these headaches of misalignment is to realign the tilts so that the muscles don't have to.

In the case of a short leg, a pad in one shoe or a specially constructed shoe may be all that is needed. The affected leg is as short as ever, but the body's tilt has been negated. A small hemipelvis can be similarly compensated for by either a slanted pillow (the thick side under the smaller bone) or a pad thick enough to lift the small side up to level with its mirror mate. Scoliosis should be medically corrected, period. The earlier the better.

Not only are the vertebrae of your spinal column overworked and underpaid (in terms of care and attention), they frequently slip a bit out of alignment. This misalignment occurs in two ways.

One way we call *subluxation*, wherein two vertebrae move slightly relative to each other. (Properly, vertebrae sit so solidly one upon the other that in essence the spinal column fits together as if it were a solid bone.) Should the first couple of vertebrae up near the skull shift slightly, a severe headache can result. You dip your head forward and pain stabs you. You stretch your neck in different positions until finally you find one that relieves the pain. The pain may constrict like a band around your head, mimicking tension headache. The subluxation problem and the pain are caused by irritation in the tough little ligaments tying the vertebrae and skull into a single unit.

A second way that vertebrae become misaligned occurs when the disks between vertebrae degenerate or slip. Then bone does not sit upon bone in your spinal column. Cartilaginous pads, called disks, between the vertebrae cushion jolts and bumps. But wear and tear takes its toll. When the pads deteriorate, flatten, or slide a little, the attendant nerves are pinched. Pinch the right nerve—that is, the wrong one—and headache results. These complex problems need to be diagnosed and treated by a physician.

The Eyes

Stanley didn't just suffer allergies. He also recently got his first pair of bifocals. Didn't he fuss and fume at his optometrist! "Ever since I got these stupid glasses, I've been getting headaches whenever I wear them! And don't tell me it's all in my head. It's the glasses!"

He was right. It was the glasses. But the prescription was not the culprit. Stanley simply wasn't used to bifocals yet. The physical work of tilting his head this way and that to focus with the appropriate lens portion was causing tension. That tension in Stanley translated into a headache.

Until Stanley got used to the two different lenses, he would get headaches from time to time. For most people, this period of adjustment, as they learn to look down through the lower part of the lens at close work then up through the upper portion at more distant objects, passes quickly.

For people who don't need glasses, eyestrain is often cited as a cause of headaches. I have found that more often it is stress and tension rather than eyestrain as such. Students with heavy loads and exams coming up may need rest, not glasses. If eyestrain is a problem for you, look at the stresses in your life first. Tend to them, and the eyestrain may go away.

A more serious source of tension headaches associated with the eyes is refractive error. That is, your eyes do not focus visual images clearly on the retina, the layer of nerve endings that sends the images to your brain. To try to compensate, you squint. Squinting causes muscle tension that can create eyestrain.

Headache associated with your eyes could also be a sign of glaucoma. Your eyeballs are water balloons of a sort. Clear fluid within them keeps them spherical. That fluid circulates through your eyes all the time; it does not just sit there, so to speak, the way water in an actual water balloon would. If any of the circulation holes plug up, blocking the flow, pressure inside the eyeball begins to build. Excessive fluid pressure on the retina kills the nerve endings there, causing blindness.

If the pressure builds slowly over time, you may have no warning of what's happening. No headache, no eye pain. Acute glaucoma, though, which occurs rapidly, zings you with a painful headache and sudden loss of vision. You need medical help immediately, but then, you knew that. Drugs can clear acute glaucoma quickly with minimum damage. To prevent damage from chronic, silent glaucoma, have your eyes examined every year or so. Make sure the examination includes a simple test for increased pressure in your eyeballs. (Doctors don't even need to touch your eye anymore; a puff of air is all it takes.)

Other Physical Anomalies

Women with ample bosoms may get headaches from wearing improperly fitted bras.

The breasts receive some support from chest and shoulder muscles. If those muscles are under a constant state of tension, and stretch, the stress can spread to the muscles higher in the shoulders where tension headaches begin. The cure is a foundation garment that draws the breasts inward and upward against the chest wall, taking some strain off the supporting muscles.

Cold Head

Cold head is a funny little phenomenon that doesn't really require a cure; it goes away in a few minutes. When susceptible persons eat a cold food such as ice cream very quickly, they sometimes experience sharp pain in their foreheads. Nibbling the food less hastily, giving it a chance to warm up a little in the mouth and throat, seems to avert the problem. Should the pain strike, the persons pause for a minute or so until the discomfort subsides, and then they can continue eating more slowly.

Teeth and Jaw

Becky was only seventeen, but already she suffered severe headaches. They didn't seem like migraines, and her family had no history of migraines. They ought to be plain old tension headaches, but she couldn't see any stresses in her life that would account for so much pain. Besides, they were more face aches than headaches and did not usually feel the way tension headaches are described. In her face and jaw in front of her ears, where the jaw hinged to the skull, is where she felt the pain most sharply. Certainly Becky knew stress firsthand; she was a high school senior with a part-time job. Still . . .

Her family dentist casually suggested that maybe she should see an orthodontist for an evaluation. No way. She adamantly refused to spend the rest of her senior year, not to mention graduation and everything, in braces. Tin teeth for the prom? Get real. Besides, the dentist didn't really insist; he merely suggested. Her dad didn't push it. Three thousand bucks?

Tin teeth in college? Becky couldn't relate to that, either. She chipped a tooth in volleyball her freshman year, however, and happened by chance to mention her headaches/faceaches to the campus dentist. He strongly recommended an orthodontist. Plagued by the nearly constant nuisance of those headaches, Becky did so.

TMJ

Becky had Temporomandibular Joint Disorder (TMJ), another of those terms Stanley would have claimed is a cop-out for healthy people who want the world to think they're sick. But it exists, it is common, and it was Becky's problem. Her teeth were crooked to the extent that her jaws did not come together properly. Her lower jaw, the mandible, could not nest into the upper jaw well enough to provide a good chewing surface. Her jaws met at only one point on each side, and the front teeth failed to meet at all by over a quarter of an inch.

When her father saw her closed-mouth X-rays, he was aghast. "I never suspected," he stammered.

"Becky is very good at hiding it," the orthodontist agreed. "I'll bet she cuts up her sandwiches into bite-size pieces and cuts the corn off roasting ears into a pile to be eaten with a fork. Because her front incisors don't come together, she can't snip food bites off or handle corn on the cob."

"I thought she was only being fastidious. Different; you know how teenagers like to think of themselves as different."

The orthodontist smiled. "Not too different. One person in five has a TMJ disorder because of jaw misalignment, but only a few get headaches from it. Poorly fitting dentures can cause it too. She's been putting up with a lot. Not only does she get headaches, but her jaw feels tender back where it hinges, and chewing hurts."

Other signs and symptoms accompany the headache. The jaw usually hurts when it's working—chewing, clenching, biting. If you get into a mouth-opening contest with other people (now there's a great pastime for the camp bunkhouse on rainy days), your jaw doesn't seem to move up and down as far as most others' do. Sometimes you can hear the joint pop or click, as if something that was hanging up suddenly broke free (which is exactly what's happening). The jaw joint in front of the ears is usually tender.

Fortunately for Becky, the orthodontist could correct her bad bite with a retaining device and a bite block worn at night. In extreme cases, jaw surgery realigns the whole bone-and-hinge complex.

With TMJ, however, I have found that there is often a nonsurgical alternative. As I work with persons suffering TMJ disorders, frequently the act of guiding them into more insight into themselves is sufficient to alleviate the discomfort. Certainly, TMJ disorders are real. Certainly at times, surgery may be required to bring the jaws into better alignment. But I find also that people blame the headaches and the facial pain on TMJ instead of their perfectionism, life stress, and personal attitudes.

If you suspect TMJ as a source of pain, go through the principles in the last few chapters before you embark on more drastic action. In short, TMJ disorders may be a fact of life, but I believe in many cases they are over-emphasized.

Abscess

Another possible headache-causing dental problem is a neglected tooth infection, or abscess.

"Well, I didn't mean to neglect it," Marcy pouted. "It just happened."

Marcy suffered a severe toothache while she was working a tight deadline at her newspaper job. She simply could not take the time to get it attended to.

Unless Marcy used analgesics heavily, she suffered pain through her jaw. More and more diffuse, it extended into her head. She could not get rid of the chronic headache until she took the time to get her abscess drained and treated. In other words, she suffered needlessly for months.

Other Dental Problems

Other dental problems can produce headaches. For example, people who grind their teeth at night (the technical term is *bruxism*) may suffer a dull, pressing headache behind the face—eyes, cheeks, forehead—when they wake up in the morning. Some doctors claim muscle tension is the culprit, and others disagree. Regardless of the cause, people who consistently grind their teeth in their sleep need dental treatment before their teeth are literally worn down and out.

I remember one case where raw recruits in an army boot camp got so mad at their instructor, clenched teeth were causing an epidemic of headache problems. As you think about sources and causes for your headaches, don't limit your ruminations to the normal, everyday considerations. It may be something interesting and unusual.

Any dental anomaly or problem can translate into a headache. If your teeth are crowded or otherwise misplaced, the way you have to compensate, even when you're not doing it consciously, can give you a headache. Make certain your dental care is up to snuff when you are evaluating possible causes for your headaches, particularly if they are persistent or chronic.

Ears

At age twelve, Benny was not yet wholeheartedly into bathing. He certainly wasn't interested in impressing girls. His mom figured he was big enough now that she shouldn't have to check him over thoroughly when he came out of the shower, and that's justifiable. He looked clean.

Benny suffered headaches near his right ear. The pain began to spread. His worried mom dragged her reluctant son to the doctor for his headaches.

Benny, it turns out, had been washing his ears by simply draping the washcloth over a finger, sticking it in his ear, and giving it a twist or two. Hey, no problem; it satisfied Mom's cursory inspection, and that's all he was interested in. His methods not only failed to clean away ear wax, they forced it back against his eardrum. It hardened there and supported a dandy colony of microbes. The irritation and infection gave him the headache.

Other ear problems can cause headaches. Fungal infections can be culprits; so is injury. Healthy ears are connected to the throat by narrow canals, the eustachian tubes. Blockage or infection in those canals can easily cause earache or headache. Here is another case where treating the headache is not as important as treating the condition causing it. The headache, which is nothing more than a symptom, will go away when the condition abates. And the condition can cause more serious problems, in this case possible hearing loss.

Neuralgias

Stanley, you will recall, just loved to complain. Every time he caught a cold (neither more nor less frequently than most people do), he complained. "I always get diseases with the word *common* in front of them. How come I never get anything really exotic; you know, like beriberi, or bilharzia, or schistosomiasis?"

His long-suffering wife stared at him. "I was wondering why you got that book on tropical diseases off the bookmobile. And now that you bring it up, bilharzia is schistosomiasis."

He glared at her. "How would you know?"

"I read the book too."

He dismissed his wife with a flap of the hand as he started to yawn. Suddenly he grimaced and took a quick breath. But it didn't seem as if he were grimacing at his wife.

Trigeminal Neuralgia

"What's wrong?" Stanley's doctor asked.

"Pain in the side of my face if I yawn too wide. It goes away in a minute or two."

"Well, Stanley!" The doctor smiled. "You may finally have something that isn't common. It's called trigeminal neuralgia, or tic douloureux. Let's run some tests."

A neuralgia is pain that runs along a nerve (*neur* meaning nerve and *algia* meaning pain). Specifically, neuralgias are sharp, stabbing pains along a nerve route which otherwise shows no physical problems—no damage, no deterioration. You will recall that the trigeminal nerve is one of the cranial nerves. A neuralgia episode begins with dull, continuous pain until a "trigger," such as a light touch, a yawn, or a breeze causes severe sharp pain, always only on one side of the face. The pain lasts from a few seconds to a minute or two. Not long, except while it's happening.

Stanley is at the young end of the scale; people under thirty-five very rarely experience trigeminal neuralgia. Incidentally, stabbing trigeminal pain in a young person (and as I get older, I consider "young" to be anything under thirty-five) should be investigated thoroughly.

The frequency of tic douloureux attacks varies. Some people experience it a couple of times a day and others very infrequently. If it occurs on the left side of the head, it will continue to strike the left side only. It does not move about or switch sides, as might migraine or other headaches.

Some people, such as Stanley, find that a particular act or touch triggers it. A man might precipitate an attack by shaving, for example, because his personal trigger point is the area on his face just over the nerve, an area sensitive to physical touch. A woman might find that she precipitates an attack by applying makeup vigorously. Stanley's trigger was wide yawning. As with other true neuralgias, this one offers no signs that something is wrong with the nerve itself.

In a goofy fifteen-second skit on the old Hee Haw television show, a patient cries, "Doctor! Doctor! I broke my arm in two places!" And the unsympathetic doctor retorts, "Then stay out of those places!"

That is essentially the treatment for your tic douloureux if you suffer the pains infrequently and your trigger point is a physical location sensitive to the touch. That is, avoid touching the area or performing the action that precipitates the attack.

I find that some patients decide not to seek treatment even though they don't know how to avoid the problem (or rather, to avoid triggering it). They opt out simply because the pain occurs too infrequently and too unpredictably to deal with.

Persons who suffer more frequent attacks generally want to do something about it. Unfortunately, there is no silver bullet. We treat trigeminal neuralgia with medication, such as carbamazepine (Tegretol). In fact, carbamazepine is a handy diagnostic tool; trigeminal neuralgia responds to it, but atypical facial pain does not, not even if it happens to occur in the area served by the trigeminal nerve. So if carbamazepine solves the problem, we can conclude that trigeminal neuralgia was the cause.

Several surgical procedures offer help for tic douloureux if all else fails. But considering the delicate nature of the trigeminal's branches, surgery is like driving in a thumbtack with a mallet. In one procedure, the nerve fibers carrying the pain are burned away with chemicals, leaving fibers which carry sensation intact. Sometimes, the patient loses feeling in the eye or in part of the face, and the numbness can be a distracting nuisance.

Advanced microsurgical procedures can reposition certain tiny blood vessels so that they squeeze the nerve. Done right, it does not cause loss of sensation, but does reduce facial pain.

Temporal Arteritis

We find temporal arteritis in elderly patients. From the name you can tell immediately that it is an inflammation *(itis)* of the arteries. It produces a headache in the temple area, just above and in front of the ears.

People suffering the problem feel weak and lose appetite. The most serious effect of temporal arteritis is loss of vision. If any vision loss accompanies the problem, you must begin treatment with steroids immediately. Promptness in treating the problem, even before it's been definitely diagnosed, may save sight, although the many available treatments vary in effectiveness.

There are a number of other neuralgias. Pain may shoot through the tongue, or the back of the mouth, or the ear. All these are treated as mentioned above, with carbamazepine, baclofen, NSAIDs, and some other drugs.

Stanley, incidentally, elected not to bother with treatment for his trigeminal neuralgia. It did not pose that great a problem for him. Besides, if his doctor did manage to fix it, he'd not be able to complain about it—or boast about it.

Pinched Nerves

Nobody who has ever experienced a pinched nerve has ever used the phrase "Oh it's only a pinched nerve." Pinched nerves are miserable, just miserable. They often cause headaches and other aches and pains.

As you get older, your bones change in important ways. They lose calcium and become less dense. They tend to bend into different shapes, which is why so many older people look hunched. The cartilaginous pads between vertebrae, the disks, flatten out and lose some of their cushioning effect. This is why you lose an inch or two in height as you get older; your spinal column's intervertebral pads are thinner. As the pads change, so does the way veterbrae sit upon one another. At the same time, the joints (especially hip joints and knees) change. The sockets wear into new shapes, and the balls and other joint ends change shape with strange new protuberances and caps of bone. Your joints may click or creak as you age.

With all this shifting and changing of the foundational bones, the nerves sometimes get caught or shifted. Most nerves lie in close association with the bones. Anything altering the bones affects them. The body has its own means for dealing with such things. The muscles around the affected bone area tighten up in an unconscious effort to "set" a broken bone or bring bones back into alignment. That muscle tension can produce its own headaches. Minor changes in neck structure, especially arthritic changes, can pinch one or more nerves and thereby cause headaches.

There's not much we can do medically about pinched nerves. Often the problem can be treated by a brief course of physical therapy, which realigns the bones and takes the pressure off. If that doesn't work, we may try medication to alleviate the pain. Don't let "getting old" be a reason to suffer needlessly.

Trauma, Concussion

A highway patrolman, Ralph made a routine car stop and pulled his vehicle, lights flashing, in behind the offender. Ralph left his vehicle and approached the other car. All routine. As Ralph leaned in through his open window on the passenger side to pick up a clipboard off the seat, a third vehicle backended his and drove it ten feet into the vehicle ahead.

Ralph never lost consciousness, but he was caught

by the doorpost and thrown. He saw and heard all that happened, but he couldn't force anything to make sense. He tried to speak and made inarticulate noises. He heard his sergeant's voice issuing orders, but could not understand them or respond.

Extensive tests revealed no physical or neurological damage whatever. And yet, for two days, Ralph's comprehension and speech periodically got all muddled. He felt dizzy. His vision blurred. He suffered almost continuous headache for several months thereafter despite treatment with narcotics and Midrin. It was some months before he could leave the temporary desk job they gave him and get back out on the road.

People assume that a head injury is going to result in a headache. Often that's true. But headache can appear any time after the incident.

Be aware too that injury to the neck and spine can also cause headaches. Any soreness in the neck muscles after a traumatic accident, or any limitation of neck movement suggests a sprain of some sort in the neck area. A throbbing headache can result, usually felt in the sides of the head. The headache may start within a week of the injury and may persist almost constantly or become periodic, and it will fade away completely in a year or two.

Only time can heal such injuries. Until time gets around to it, try the usual analgesics for tension headache first, before graduating if necessary to medication. In the case of a neck injury, or whiplash, try hot packs on the neck and over-the-counter pain relievers. If that doesn't provide relief, the next level of attack is nonsteroidal antiinflammatory drugs and possible steroids or combinations of medications.

Now and then, a violent injury to the head or neck marks the beginning of migraine, cluster headaches, or tension headaches in people who did not have that sort of thing before the injury occurred. These secondary headaches could be caused by the stress of an accident, by some physical damage (although very rarely does an actual physical cause ever show up), or by the emotional jolt of a traumatic injury. Sometimes we have no idea why they occur.

Air Pressure Change

Do you get a headache when a hurricane blows through? You sure can. The triggering mechanism is a sudden drop in barometric pressure. This change in turn messes up your arteries' attempts to keep your blood pressure even and ideal. A lot of people get headaches during severe storms. It's not just tension. It's physical.

You should look out for another situation regarding barometric pressure change, especially in the west: altitude sickness. That can give you a zinger of a headache. Picture yourself standing at the bottom of a vertical column of air that stretches from the ground beneath your feet to the top of the atmosphere. The weight of that vertical column of air is always pushing on you in all directions (yes, air has weight). Your body automatically compensates for that pressure; in fact, your arteries use it as they dilate or retract to control your blood pressure. Also, delicate nuances of pressure dictate how well your blood transports oxygen and carbon dioxide.

Since the atmosphere forms a fairly uniform skin

over the earth's surface, by and large, if you walk around at sea level, you have about the same weight of air on you at all times. But as you climb a high mountain, you have less and less air above you as you go. Less weight; less pressure. In a word, as you go up in elevation, the air pressure becomes less. Airplanes compensate for this by pressurizing the cabin as they gain elevation.

Your arteries are used to your normally-lived-in elevation. Let's say you are accustomed to 1000 feet elevation. Should you drive over the Sierras through Yosemite National Park, you will rise rapidly to 9000 feet elevation—and stay there a while. In their frantic bid to compensate for the sudden change, your arteries may respond by giving you a severe headache.

How then do mountain climbers cope with altitude sickness? They rise in elevation slowly, over a period of days, letting their bodies adjust by stages. They train for a while at 10,000 feet or so, go up a few thousand feet, spend a day or two, then ascend further. By the time they're ready for the final assault to, say, 22,000 feet, their bodies are accustomed to the thin air. But some people simply cannot tolerate higher elevations and still get altitude sickness no matter how slowly they climb.

Altitude sickness does not work in reverse. People who live at high elevations don't have problems descending to the heavier pressure of lower elevations.

Infections and Metabolic Problems

Much as I dislike seeing lists in books, I'd like to give you a brief list of infectious diseases and other problems that may cause headaches. As you are considering your own headache problem, skim this list and consult your doctor if you suspect one of the items on it may be a contributing factor.

- Diabetes (characterized by severe thirst, abnormal hunger, and frequent urination)
- Sexually-transmitted infections such as herpes, syphillis, AIDS
- Tuberculosis (chest pain, cough, and weakness)
- Influenza virus
- Anything with fever as a symptom
- Anoxia (situation in which lack of oxygen causes problems)
- Aneurisms and hemorrhage (especially if you have high blood pressure)
- Stroke (sudden paralysis, speech or memory problems)
- Lupus (an auto-immune disease indicated by lumps in the skin, joint pain, and rash)
- Other viral infections—mumps, mononucleosis, yellow fever, Dengue fever, and others
- Other bacterial diseases—pneumonia, kidney infections, and Lyme disease may involve a headache. So, too, do strange and exotic illnesses we don't hear much about, such as anthrax, brucellosis, tetanus, plague, tularemia, typhoid, etc.
- A recent lumbar puncture. In about a third of patients, the puncture itself can cause a headache lasting up to several days. Pain will be dull or throbbing, aggravated by erect posture, and relieved by lying down.

The list is not complete, but you can see the general idea. Always, always take conditions such as these into consideration as you discuss your problems with your doctor.

Your average healthy kid sometimes seems accident prone. I remember many a time when one of my own children crashed while horseback riding or got instantly sick for, it seemed, no reason at all. Every parent knows the feeling of personal hurt as the beleaguered child sobs a request to be held and cosseted. There is nothing you can do at first, really, to allay the pain except to hold and to soothe and perhaps to kiss the booboo.

Children present special concerns, and yes, they do indeed get headaches, including migraines. Let us look at their special needs next.

CHAPTER 13

Headaches in Kids

Eleven-year-old Greg wasn't a bad kid. He was a good reader, with his nose in a book all the time. Unfortunately, his fertile young mind discovered in books a lot of nifty ideas that adults didn't find all that funny. For example, after reading about some pranks described in the reminiscences of an English schoolboy (a really old book, incidentally), he glued a half dollar to the head of a galvanized masonry nail. He drove the nail into a crack in the sidewalk so that the half dollar "lay" on the cement. From the house, he videotaped people spotting the half dollar and trying unsuccessfully to pick it up. The prank kept him amused for days. Unfortunately, one of the subjects on his video threatened his dad with a lawsuit.

Greg's dad, understandably, suffered more than one headache because of Greg's antics. But Greg, too, experienced occasional headaches. They could come at any time, but usually they happened on Fridays. They lasted four or five hours.

At first Greg's mother refused to believe him. "Kids don't have headaches," she insisted. "You're just saying that to get out of cleaning your room. So how about cutting out the nonsense and getting started on this pigpen?"

When his complaints persisted, his mom took him to the optometrist. "He reads too much," she insisted. "Eyestrain." The optometrist found no problems with Greg's eyes and no need for corrective lenses.

Wisely, she was afraid to give Greg aspirin. "I forget what they call it," she told a neighbor, "but it's a disease that can happen if kids take aspirin. Do you think Tylenol would be safe?"

She took him to the pediatrician. The doctor could find nothing physically wrong. Long familiar with Greg and his ways, the physician suggested a psychological evaluation.

"Nonsense! He's all boy, but he's not nuts!" Still, as Greg's mom thought about it, he did seem a little strange sometimes. And he really did seem to be suffering with headaches, as he claimed. It grated on her immensely to have to put off cleaning the house one Monday morning—she always cleaned on Fridays and Mondays—but she took Greg to a psychologist.

Greg and his mom illustrate several points of which you should be aware.

If Kids Really Get Headaches, Are They Serious?

Greg's mom had always heard that kids don't suffer headaches like adults do.

Says Dr. Paul Warren, behavioral pediatrician at the Minirth Meier New Life Clinics, "Headaches really do occur in the lives of kids. We've found a probable incidence of from four to ten percent of kids suffering from true vascular headaches such as migraine. Unfortunately, headaches can be happening and you don't know it."

Children, particularly young ones, usually cannot articulate the pain and problems they feel. "It hurts, Mommy," is not a very helpful analysis. (Sometimes Mommy doesn't even get that much to work with.)

Children with a headache will be fussy, out of sorts, crying and whining a lot. They may hold their heads with their hands, press on their temples, or snuggle in and keep their heads very, very still. Think about the nonverbal things you do when you get a headache. Now translate that into actions your small child might take. Do the actions you see suggest headache?

Older children are normally a little better at explaining what they feel. One young man we interviewed described the pain: "It's like someone tying a shoelace around your head real tight." Not only eloquent, his description was useful too.

Yes, But Is My Child's Headache Dangerous?

"Usually, headaches in children arise from a cold or allergy," says Dr. Warren. "They aren't all that uncommon. Persistent headaches, though, should be a concern. They may be manifestations of depression or fear, or, in very rare cases, a serious physical problem. If a high fever and vomiting accompany a headache, seek evaluation immediately. I do mean immediately."

"When you say immediately, you scare the willies out of me!" moans Greg's mom.

When we raise the spectre of serious problems, we

never mean to frighten anyone. But we do mean to inform. The possibility that your child's headache is the harbinger of some life-threatening illness is remote at best. But under certain circumstances a neurologist should check the child, just to be safe.

What are some of the conditions a neurologist should look for?

Life-Threatening Conditions

Brain tumors. Headaches are usually a late symptom of tumors, in children as well as adults. Were a tumor to grow on your elbow, it would have plenty of room to expand outward. You would notice a bigger and bigger lump. But tumors growing within the head have nowhere to go. As they grow they exert increasing pressure on whatever part of the brain they lie next to. Logically, you look for signs that some part of the brain isn't operating up to snuff: memory lapses, tingling or reduced function in an arm or leg, mood changes, changes in speech. We are talking, of course, about unusual changes rather than the normal changes kids undergo as they grow up. Brain tumors do occur in children, but they are exceedingly rare.

Headaches caused by tumors typically occur rather late in the game. When they do, they may be particularly strong in the morning as the child first gets up, and they are often accompanied by vomiting.

Infections. Encephalitis is an infection of parts of the head. Meningitis germs affect the meninges, the delicate membranes encasing the nervous system. Both illnesses present symptoms in addition to headache, but headache is a part of it. They do occur with some frequency in kids.

Because aspirin can cause Reye's Syndrome, a very serious illness, don't pop an aspirin into a sick child. If your child complains of a headache along with vague flulike symptoms, call a physician immediately. And always use an aspirin substitute. Tylenol is fine.

Vascular malformation. Sometimes problems with an artery or other blood vessel in the head can cause headaches. Your physician will use an MRI, CAT scan, or other test to evaluate the situation.

Major Trauma. A child with a headache who has been involved in an accident should be evaluated by a physician immediately, particularly a child with a concussion. Also, children with post brain injury—that is, kids who were hurt and now are recovering—may suffer a lot of headaches.

Head injuries are especially common in toddlers. They have large heads and weak necks compared to older children and adults, so heads get bumped more. Too, their lack of coordination sends them lurching and tumbling constantly.

Other Childhood Illnesses

Many illnesses of childhood, some of which are accompanied by headaches, are neither dangerous nor life-threatening:

So-called eyestrain. Greg's mom was in error when she attributed headaches to eyestrain as such. Eyestrain per se does not usually cause headaches. But too much reading might cause problems in another way. Kids who bunch up in weird positions as they read can conceivably get tension headaches if their muscles knot.

Also, uncorrected vision problems can cause headaches. The child's eye muscles tighten up, trying to compensate for lens defects, and the resulting tension causes a headache. Greg's mom was wise to take him to an optometrist.

Glaucoma is a disease causing raised fluid pressure within the eyeball. If it is left untreated, the continual pressure on the retina eventually causes blindness. Simple tests quickly identify the presence of glaucoma, and everyone, child and adult alike, should be tested periodically.

Sinuses. The multitude of childhood ear, nose, and throat ailments can sometimes cause headaches. So can sinus infections and allergies, but rarely.

Where to Go for Help

Greg's mom first took her son to the pediatrician and to the optometrist, both good moves. A family practice specialist is an excellent first step also.

Chronic, persistent headaches call for evaluation by a neurologist as a second step. Assuming the neurologist finds no physical cause for the headaches, it is time to look toward a psychological source.

"Let me caution against the phrase 'It's all in your head,'" says Dr. Warren. "I dislike the term *psychosomatic* because of the connotations. It suggests that the pain is false, that the child is somehow faking it. That's not true. The pain, whatever its source, is very real. For that reason I prefer the term *psychophysiological*, which does not carry a connotation of faking.

"When we tell a kid, 'There's nothing going on; it's all in your head,' we may be telling the truth in the purest sense. But we thereby lose the opportunity to help the kid learn how to cope with the headache. We lose the opportunity to find out what's going on inside the kid that's causing it. Either of those two opportunities is infinitely more important than gaining an empty point for truth."

Psychological evaluation. Greg's mom grimaced at the thought. She wasn't at all sure that Greg's symptoms were serious enough to warrant the trouble and expense of a psychologist. To evaluate how much headaches, plus whatever they are accompanying, are affecting a child, ask three questions (the questions assume physicians found no physical cause):

1. Do headaches affect how the child functions socially? How does the child get along with family, teachers, peers? Do the headaches limit or curtail social activities?
2. Do the headaches alter other ways in which the child relates to his or her world? How are sports, recess, and other activities affected? Is schoolwork okay? Does the child lose enthusiasm for hobbies, reading, and other personal interests?
3. Is the child in obvious discomfort?

Greg's mom ended up saying "yes" to several of those items, so she chose a psychologist who routinely worked with kids and had a good reputation for dealing with them. That selectively was another wise move.

She had never been to a psychologist before. She had never dreamed she might be dragging Greg off to one. As she stepped into the woman's office for the first time, she muttered aloud, "What in the world am I getting myself into?"

What she was getting into was the beginning of the solution to Greg's headaches and her frequent ones as well.

Treating Headaches in Kids

Actually, as Greg's mom thought about it, this wasn't nearly as bad as she envisioned. The room in which the psychologist conducted this initial interview was appointed more like a living room than an office, with pretty, overstuffed chairs and a sofa, color-coordinated carpets and draperies, walnut end tables, and lamps that did not look like they came out of a cheap motel. That was Greg's mom's major complaint with most doctors' offices: the lamps were usually so ugly.

The psychologist herself, Mrs. Brubaker, probably approaching thirty-five, looked crisp and well groomed without appearing stiff or cold. Greg's mom admired that.

Mrs. Brubaker directed a lot of her questions to Greg's mom, not to him. That seemed odd. Just now she was asking about Greg's mom's housecleaning. Perhaps she was seeking some pointers.

"I go through the house on Friday to make certain it's ready for the weekend. Then on Monday I give it a thorough cleaning. You know what a weekend will do to a house."

"Oh, my, yes. Trash time." Mrs. Brubaker smiled at Greg. "Do you help with housework?"

"No, ma'am."

It pleased Greg's mom that her kid was remembering his manners. She added, "I tried teaching him; you know, vacuuming and that. But he drove me crazy. Lackadaisical. Never did it thoroughly or right. So I just make him clean up his room. Even that can take him all evening. Pick up some clothes, get his books and things in order, and it takes him all evening."

Mrs. Brubaker nodded sagely. "A place for everything and everything in its place."

"Oh, absolutely!" Greg's mom could see this woman was on her wavelength, all the way.

Mrs. Brubaker smiled at Greg. She did a lot of smiling, and it all looked sincere. "Greg, there's a stack of books and things in the next room there. Would you excuse us a few minutes, please, while we check schedules?" She nodded toward a side door.

It took Greg a moment to catch on. He mumbled, "Sure," and left through the door.

The door barely clicked shut before Greg's mom asked nervously, "Do you know what's happening? Have you learned anything?"

"Perhaps so. You mentioned you suffer from tension headaches. They are not uncommon in the kids I see, either. They are happening in Greg. They hurt; and they are happening for reasons we can't measure with tests. So we do two things: we use an analgesic to get rid of the immediate pain—you're doing this when you give him Tylenol—and we look for long-term conflict or stress that is causing the problem."

"Headaches are a symptom, not a disease. I know."

Mrs. Brubaker turned on her radiant smile. "Right! Now, we can set up a series of sessions, or we can try an experiment in behavior modification—a one-shot thing, you might say. Are you game?"

"Behavior modification? Yes, let's. Greg can certainly use some."

"Not Greg. You."

And suddenly Greg's mom was not at all sure this woman knew what she was doing. "We're here for Greg's headaches."

Mrs. Brubaker nodded.

"Are you saying I'm causing his headaches by being firm with him or something?"

"Let's see. How can I put this?" Mrs. Brubaker ruminated a few moments. "Two points. One: We think that sometimes kids learn from their family system— all this below the conscious level, understand—that headaches are the way you deal with stress. Two: Greg's headaches usually occur on Fridays, occasionally on Mondays, and hardly ever at any other time. Did you notice?"

"I notice they're terribly convenient when it comes time for him to clean up his room or do the dishes."

"Might he not be finding those particular times stressful?"

"Stressful!? He doesn't do a blooming thing. Except clean up his room, which is what he's supposed to be doing anyway."

"To your standard of excellence, not his."

Greg's mom wrinkled her nose. "He doesn't have one."

"My point. Here's the experiment I suggest: For the next four weekends, totally ignore the condition of his room. Don't make an issue of it; don't even tell him to clean it up. I guarantee that this will drive you right out of your tree. It will take a herculean effort on your part to remain silent. After the four weeks, establish a minimum standard that he must observe only if and when you have house guests."

"How minimum?"

"No drawers hanging open, all clothes either in the hamper or hidden in the closet—"

"He'd pile them on the closet floor."

"So be it. We're talking minimal. No furniture tipped over. All shoes under the bed. Let's make an appointment three weeks from today to evaluate his headache problem further. He may well have other sources of excessive stress in his life; we don't want to miss any possible causes. This is just an experiment."

Greg's mom reluctantly agreed. To her amazement, Greg's mom saw almost immediate improvement in her son. No headaches, no complaints. She was not amazed to observe that she herself just about went crazy over that room. She had to leave the house to keep from running in there and putting it in order herself.

They held five sessions in all, Greg and his mom and Mrs. Brubaker. By the end of the series, Greg's mom was reevaluating her own standards for housekeeping. She found herself able to let Greg be a kid once in a while and even taught him how to cook breakfasts he liked despite the fact that he made a royal mess in the kitchen.

Greg's mom used to get headaches three or four times a week. Now they come maybe once a month. And Greg? No headaches at all.

Vascular Headaches in Children

The situation with Greg and his mom was more complex than this little narrative suggests. Changing a few behaviors was not a magic bullet to make everything all right. There were other issues, other factors, and Greg's dad took part in the subsequent sessions as well. The primary aim was to get the family sitting down and talking to each other.

"When a child complains of a headache, and especially if the child complains frequently, don't just assume it's a ploy of some sort. Pay attention," Dr. Warren advises. "Think of it as a caution flag. An alert. Get the child to talk about it. Where and when? What is it like? And always keep in mind that the child is not an independently functioning person the way an adult is. The child is a close adjunct of the family and is influenced far more by the family than is an adult."

The most common diagnoses we find at the emotional level are anxiety and depression, frequent causes of persistent headaches in kids, and they are not easily alleviated. You will want professional help in dealing with them. You will want professional help, too, if your child is one of those unfortunate kids who suffers migraine.

What you've learned about migraines in adults pretty much applies to kids as well. Doctors look for a family history of migraines. They also look for certain personality types. In youngsters, we often find that migraine sufferers are bright, smart, verbal, and probably obsessive about some things. They are usually firstborns. However, not all children who suffer headaches, by any means, fit into those types. The most casual, easygoing child can be a migraine sufferer.

The headaches can occur on one side or on both. Frequently, they are preceded by some prodromal phenomenon, an aura. If the children can explain how they feel, they say that things happen. They get a strange feeling or a sick feeling. They may become nauseous during the warning phase. They may see flickering or flashing lights before and during the headache.

Children locked into the misery of one of these headaches desire most of all to simply go to sleep. After some hours of rest, they seem to have slept it off, and they feel much better.

Migraines and tension headaches are not life-threatening, of course, but they may feel that way to the child. Is there hope for a headache-free adulthood for the 10 percent or so of children who get them?

These kids are at high risk in that they will need a physician's care into adulthood. And yet, not all kids who suffer tension headaches and migraine in childhood get them in later life. It is not a sure sentence to a lifetime of pain. As children get older, their headaches should be treated appropriately according to their age and level of maturity.

The pain of headaches, even low-level tension headaches, is very distracting and discouraging for children. They've not been conditioned yet to understand that headaches can be expected, as have adults. They find themselves throwing temper tantrums they don't really want to throw, getting into trouble they didn't really intend to get into, missing schoolwork when they know they can do better. The irritation of the headaches is compounded by irritation at themselves for such poor performance.

Because of this and because kids' function is reduced significantly, parents have to be aggressive in treating their kids' headaches.

If we as adults don't help kids with headaches, we find the kids may begin to medicate themselves. They'll use aspirin, alcohol, marijuana, whatever folk medicines other kids suggest. Not yet enured to headaches, the kids will find some way out of them. Needless to say, an inappropriate cure can be far worse than the headache.

Extreme Cases

Greg's case was mild, a tension headache put to rights by adjusting home life somewhat (not an easy adjustment for either him or his mom, but do-able). At the other extreme on the spectrum, we find ourselves dealing with kids who are out of control both physically and emotionally.

Certainly we must find out why those children's behaviors and headaches are occurring, but we must also provide a safe environment in which to turn them around. We have to protect the kids from themselves and from their situations. Sometimes that protection cannot be achieved while the children are home. To that end, we may need to put children in a structured environment where we can evaluate them and closely control the medications that they need. Usually, the structured environment is a hospital of some sort.

The vast majority of hurting children don't need this. But those who do, need it desperately.

For children and adults both, medication should be considered a stopgap and, whenever possible, a last resort. Genuine relief from headaches means being relieved from their ravages altogether, not beating them down with a stick after they attack. This requires a three-pronged approach, healing body, mind, and spirit.

I want to devote the next two chapters to exploring solutions which move beyond medicine to mend the complete fabric of the headache sufferer's life. Medication—popping a couple of aspirin or committing to a lifetime drug regimen—is strictly second best to true and lasting relief.

Kids and adults alike can master headaches. Not just reduce them but master them. Throughout this book we have been offering principles and guidelines. Here and there, as we discussed different types of headaches, we've talked about the medications and other steps the headache sufferer can take to find relief. Now it is time to discuss the effective steps people can take which do not require medication. They are more effective and more lasting than any medications can be.

Let us put those principles together now into a concise arrangement, a guide for the person who would find freedom from pain.

CHAPTER 14

The Seven-Pronged Cure, Part I: Body and Mind

You certainly wouldn't call Melody a weird hippie throwback to the 60s. She was a weird hippie throwback to the 60s, but you wouldn't call her that because her husband Gus was six feet four, weighed 260 pounds—none of it fat—and could bench press a Shetland pony. Gus was very protective of Melody. So you call her "particular about what her family eats," if you call her anything at all, and let it go at that.

Melody, Gus, and their children ingested none but fertilized brown eggs, no bread except cracked wheat ground in Melody's own handmill, no factory-processed foods whatsoever. If Melody could have, she would have prevented her family from being tainted with smog and other chemicals by forbidding them all to breathe. To say that Melody obsessed about unnatural chemicals was putting it mildly.

There was one situation, however, when she was forced to submit to artificial chemicals in a big way: when she suffered her frequent tension headaches, and Gus was struck down by major migraine. Then they had to pop maximum allowable quantities of prescription painkillers. Over-the-counter medications wouldn't do the job. In fact, in Gus's case, not even heavy-duty prescription medications made a dent in his misery. Eventually such headaches became chronic and habitual.

"I just don't understand," she moaned. "There's absolutely no reason for us to get these vicious headaches. No chemicals or preservatives. Wholesome diet. Clean country air. We subsistence farm, you know. We raise all our own food except citrus. We live a peaceful rural existence with no tensions and hassles."

Few persons can make that claim these days. Certainly, Agatha Wier could not. Aggie worked at a metropolitan newspaper on the city desk. She lived a tension-laden life under more daily stress than most of us. She experienced constant deadlines, heavy political pressure, meals on the run, guilt, and frantic activity as she tried to balance her work against her home life and teenage kids. And yet, Aggie suffered very few headaches.

Life-style alone neither condemns you to headaches nor releases you from them. Aggie managed her headaches by applying eight principles that will work for you also as you deal with your own headache problems.

To begin with, you must realize what Aggie learned: You have to treat the whole person, body, mind, and spirit, not just the headache. Any specific recommendations that I make all point toward that end, whether or not they seem to. The whole person.

Managing headaches is always second best to preventing them. The first principle, then, is to avoid headaches when possible.

Our first four prongs of treatment (some of which I have mentioned earlier) will deal with your body and mind. The last three prongs deal with your mind and spirit.

1. Prevention

Gus and Melody ended up talking to me about headaches by default, so to speak. They were friends of friends.

Gus seemed particularly angry. "We avoid alcohol. We certainly don't smoke. We avoid stress. This shouldn't be happening!"

I let that one by for the moment and got them talking about horses. You see, I love horses. So do my girls. We'll go out riding just about every weekend, either merely messing around or doing something organized with the horses—a gymkhana or something. Gus and Melody know a great deal about horses, so for the next ten minutes, the conversation flowed fast and fun.

It was time for me to bring the conversation around to headaches again. "Great stress reliever, out riding."

Gus grinned. "Sure is."

"Of course, the horses can be a problem, too. I remember when Alicia's pony mare went lame. Alicia's too young to understand what was happening; 'sore foot' was about the extent of it. She still doesn't know we almost lost that horse—that we almost had to put it down. And the stringhalt in Rachel's favorite really bothered us. Stringhalt doesn't ruin a horse, but it spoils it for showing."

"I hear you." Gus's light mood darkened a little. "We lost a good horse last month. Twisted gut. You know how bad that can be."

I nodded. Perfectly good, healthy horses can get sick and die in a day if their intestinal tracts become so looped or everted that the tissues die. It doesn't happen often, but it happens.

Melody added, "And last winter we had to put down a yearling that got tangled in barbed wire." She scowled. "It wasn't even our fencing. We won't allow barbed wire on our property because of the horses. The little gelding got out—he was an escape artist anyway—and stepped into loose fencing coils down at the neighbor's. Really tore him up."

"I'd guess it really tore you up too. Emotionally, I mean."

"Yeah, it did. That was a good horse."

The Seven-Pronged Attack on Headaches

1. Prevention
2. Home remedies without use of drugs
3. Diet manipulation to control headaches
4. Medications, non-prescription and prescription
5. Insight into personality and feelings
6. Cognitive restructuring—thinking along new lines
7. New behavior—to change the innermost feelings that actually control us

---

On our farm we don't keep horses only. We have just about every other kind of farm animal as well, even a llama. So I could talk to Gus and Melody with some familiarity about chickens and hogs and sheep. In the next three minutes, as we discussed the dangers and illnesses that befall animals, Melody nearly came to tears.

It became clear that they both took a deep personal interest in every animal on their farm. They knew them all, even the sheep, which you would think all look alike. Melody got some of her worst headaches in autumn. She attributed it to allergy. Goldenrod. She could be right; goldenrod might have been a factor. But having talked to her, I strongly doubted that was the primary cause.

Fall, you see, is butchering time.

Your Prevention Checklist

Most likely, you do not do much butchering. But Melody had totally discounted that source of stress and sorrow by failing to recognize it as such. Deep grieving was involved here. And yet, as she later pointed out, what could she do about it? I suggested having the butchering done elsewhere. A large part of the stress was having to do it herself.

Curiously enough, that did help. She and Gus sent their meat animals off to a neighbor's to be slaughtered, cut, and wrapped; out of sight, out of (immediate) mind. In return, the neighbor had Melody and Gus prepare his winter meat for him. It didn't bother her nearly so much to render animals to which she held no special attachment. A bonus: She does excellent work, and she was justly proud of the job they did for the neighbor. She'd never before been able to show off her talents, so to speak.

As you are assaying ways to prevent headaches, therefore, think about what displeases or upsets you. Could be a source. As you study possible stress sources, think also about how to allay them, at least partially, as Melody did.

The first step in headache prevention then is:

- Allay stress sources. Either avoid them or deal with them.

Secondly:

- Get appropriate sleep.

People's sleep needs vary greatly. Children in particular often fail to get sufficient rest. That one step, which is also a sound investment in overall health, can make a big difference.

Next:

- Try to eat on a regular schedule.

A friend of mine says, "Our kids are in their teens, and my husband works odd hours. Breakfast is staggered, no one is home at lunch, and dinner could be crazy. So we adopted supper. The nutritionists say you shouldn't eat a heavy meal late in the evening, so I cook light. But it's a full meal. We all sit at the table. We eat with formal place settings and candlelight. Appetizer is tomato juice or orange juice. Yes, it's that formal.

"If the kids think they absolutely must see something that's on TV then, they have to tape it to watch afterwards. The whole idea is to have one relaxed meal together in the day. No rushing, just conversation. I thought for a while that I was perhaps forcing the kids into doing something they hated; you know, raising their stress level. No such thing. They look forward to it now."

She frowned. "And Beth doesn't get her morning headaches so much anymore. Do you think the reduced stress is it?"

Regular meals promote uniform blood sugar levels. The routine greatly reduces stress also, particularly for kids. They thrive on regularity and routine. In the midst of this, however, remember these principles too:

- Avoid overeating.
- Avoid smoking.
- Avoid alcohol.
- Exercise in moderation.

"Fat chance," grumbled Gus. "A subsistence farm is constant work, most of it involving strenuous exercise. You plow fields, weed the garden, drive cows from here to there, chop stovewood. Moderation? No way."

I am talking here primarily to the person who does not exercise much during the routine of the day or who exercises infrequently and tries to make up for four slack days in one. Gus's stamina and muscles were well toned. He was accustomed to strenuous daily activity. Exercise shouldn't be a big headache source for him, or for you if you have a physical job as well.

In addition:

- Stay on top of health problems.

This advice makes sense in itself, of course. Whether you discover a major malady—diabetes or such—or some minor health annoyance—a toothache, perhaps—prompt attention will minimize ill effects. Don't let it drag along, as do many who feel they are too busy or (let's face it) too lazy to take care of it immediately. This will also minimize resulting headaches and prevent complications. Make health care a priority, headaches or no.

• Modify your behavior.

I love this quote by William James: "The Lord may forgive us our sins, but the nervous system never does." Behavior modification forgives the physical.

Melody sniffed. "We don't have any behavior that needs modifying." At first glance, she would appear to be right. But then we looked again. Here was a typical day for this lady who led a stress-free, bucolic existence:

• Up at four-thirty to milk, feed the calves, do early chores
• Get the kids up at six and off to school (a major hassle; they had over an hour bus ride)
• When they get home, supervise their chores, homework
• Feed chickens, hogs, horses; tend vegetable garden, lawn, flower beds, orchard, five acres of Christmas trees
• Start bread rising (food preparation consumed three hours daily at least)
• Housework, laundry, and all that

- Help Gus with machinery repair, field work (mostly seasonal but demanding; you have to plow now, cultivate the corn now, combine the wheat now when it's ready, not when you get to it), animal care such as shoeing horses, dehorning calves ad infinitum
- Handle seasonal loads: lambing, pig farrowing, county fair time, Christmas, etc.
- Milking, twice a day, every day
- For extra money, sew items such as dolls, quilts, and braided rugs to be sold on commission through several gift shops
- Read to the kids, interact with them, be a mom; take them to athletic events and practices, ferry them back and forth to all the after-school and extracurricular things kids get into (going to town was a forty minute drive each way)
- Be a wife and lover

And those were the good times, the easy days. When a child or animal got sick, not to mention when harvest and canning and freezing rolled around, or when plowing and planting took priority, her stress multiplied exponentially. Melody lived in an idyllic rural setting, but she never ever got to sit. The closest she could come to relaxing was sitting under the apple tree shelling peas or doing the handwork on a gift item. Melody's life was as constantly busy and stressful as was Aggie's. Aggie saw her situation and took steps to counter it. But Melody, by failing to recognize the pressure, did nothing about it.

Melody sagged, defeated. "The healthy life-style is very important to Gus and me both, and especially for the kids' sake. Now you're telling me it's not healthy for me. But it's what we want! My life's not always that hectic. You're overstating the situation."

"When is the last time you took a vacation?"

"You don't take a vacation when there's two cows to milk."

"When is the last full week when nothing went wrong, such as illness, major equipment breakdown, or emergencies?"

"Why, just last . . . uh . . . ." She grimaced. "But I can't change any of that. I don't want to."

I nodded. "Then you must change. That's where behavior modification comes in."

Behavior Modification

On the outside of a clever Thanksgiving greeting card I saw some years ago, a cartoon turkey stands on a soapbox with one "finger" pinion raised, a pose of pontification. Inside it says, "You are what you eat." So true. Melody would be the first to agree, which is why she worked so hard to provide her family wholesome food. This statement is also true: "You are what you do."

Behavior modification is not visualization. Persons who have success in other areas using visualization techniques may want to try them with headache management as well. Behavior modification, however, is a somewhat different breed of cat.

The basis of behavior modification is twofold. First, if you want to change the way you think or feel, you do the things that promote those thoughts and feelings. It is essentially the reverse of the dictum you already know, that your thoughts and feelings affect how you act.

This reversal works well. By acting according to the thoughts and feelings you want to promote, they come. Just as thoughts control your actions, your mind responds to the physical cues your body sends.

You know that if you dwell on certain thoughts long enough, they affect you. For example, in 2 Samuel, David, King of Israel, committed adultery with the wife of Uriah, getting her pregnant. He became obsessed with removing Uriah to cover their sin. It nearly destroyed him even before God called him to account and severely judged him.

On the other hand, even in the darkest adversity, as Saul was trying to kill him, he had lost his wife Michal, and his doom seemed assured, David never ceased blessing and praising God. However sorrowful he might feel, he sang of his joy and trust in his Lord. Though practically speaking he had no cause for joy, he adopted it anyway, and it never ceased to buoy him up. In the aftermath of the Uriah affair, when his life lay in shambles, he praised his Lord and could again step forth boldly.

Do you feel happy? You will enjoy pleasant things. Do you feel sad and want to feel happier? Do pleasant things. The happy feelings follow.

That is one face of behavior modification. The other is using changes in external behavior to solve internal problems that hamper you and rob you of the happiness God intended for you.

Melody's problem was dealing with the constant galloping busyness, stress, and tensions of her everyday life. She could not remove the factors causing the stress. She had to alter her reactions, in this case, shedding tension. And there is where behavior modification—exactly the techniques Aggie used to good advantage in the city—came to Melody's aid.

Try for yourself this behavioral exercise Aggie used, and I suggested to Melody ("I can't afford the time," Melody wailed. "You can't afford not to," I countered):

- Sit in a comfortable, relaxing easy chair such as a recliner or old rocker. Ideally, its back is high enough to support your head.
- Take a deep, deep breath, hold it a moment, and release it all at once. Close your eyes.
- Concentrate on your hands and arms. Tighten every muscle there. Clench your fists! Now, paying attention to those tensed muscles, relax them instantly, as if dropping the tension out a second story window. When you think they're relaxed, loosen them more. Let your arms lie flaccid for at least half a minute.
- Concentrate on your legs and toes. Again, tighten all the muscles, making opposing muscles work against each other. (This will take some practice. You'll get good enough at it that every muscle will be straining and your legs won't move a millimeter.) Relax them. More. Flaccid.
- Do the same with trunk muscles. Tuck in your neck. Suck in your stomach! Washboard stomach like Gus's? Suck it in anyway. Relax.
- Finally, do the same with your face and the neck muscles serving your jaw. Relax. Your jaw should drop open spontaneously. Your face should look dull and emotionless.

When your face has been thus relaxed for thirty seconds or so, stop and think about what you've been thinking. As you began the exercise you may well have been pondering the next crisis or responsibility of the busy day. When you finish, if the relaxation has been nearly total (your muscles never relax completely unless you're dead), your mind will be relatively free of frantic thought.

Melody spent five minutes at this exercise following lunch and another five near the close of day.

Look over the graphs supplied earlier in the book. See how many headaches mention muscle tension as a contributing factor. Anything you do to reduce stress and relax tension can do no harm in these cases, and just might help greatly.

The important lesson in Melody's life, and yours, is that tension must be identified before it can be eliminated. When it is, headache incidence will abate.

2. Home Remedies

"Home remedies? Herbs! Natural remedies! Wonderful!" Melody waxed enthusiastic instantly. Clearly she expected me to give her a list of plants to graze.

"External remedies," I amended.

The only remedy for Gus's migraines, and it did very little to actually curtail the headaches, was to rest in a darkened room. Melody, however, had some excellent options for cutting her tension headaches short, options that work for more than just tension headaches, some of which I mentioned earlier.

- Lie down in a warm bath. The warm water makes certain adjustments in your vascular system that may ease or even altogether relieve the problem.

- Try using a cool cloth on your head. This works for some people and not for others. It's certainly worth experimenting with.
- Massage the neck and shoulders, particularly the muscles where neck and shoulder join.

Some people claim that certain herbal teas, such as chamomile, aid headaches. I can't recommend herbal teas because they vary so much as to content, not just between blends but within blends. You really do not know what you're getting in them.

"I know what I'm getting in my chamomile tea," Melody snaps. "All chamomile and nothing but. I raise my own chamomile out by the back stoop. It's a beautiful little bush with white daisylike flowers."

"I'm sure your chamomile is unadulterated. But we still can't say what's in it. The chemicals vary too much by season and region to be predictable."

I'm not saying don't try herbals. By all means do. But don't expect them to work in you the way they work in your friend who recommended them—or in Melody, for that matter. Find what works for you. And keep in mind that even "safe" herbs and teas can cause adverse reactions in others—perhaps you. Pay attention to your body as you experiment.

You understand by now, I think, that everything you ingest, be it food or drink, contains chemicals. Complex chemicals. That is why diet is so important.

3. Diet

I already made diet suggestions when we were discussing migraines. Headache sufferers of all types ought to try them. They are detailed in chapter five.

I might mention one other aspect of diet that you might consider. A friend of mine claims that he has no allergies or dietary flukes as such, but his digestion gets into trouble if he loads too many different kinds of foods into it. The variety nails him, he says, with mild headache, indigestion, and loose bowels. He first noticed it when he joined a church that loved to eat (don't we all!) and began attending innumerable potlucks for various occasions. He thought at first he got a touch of food poisoning from someone's improperly cooled casserole or something, but no one else experienced any problems. When he limited his potluck forays to one or two offerings per supper, the problem disappeared.

There it is again: paying attention to your body.

4. Medications

When a man named Michael could not shake his obsessions, he was sent to me. I'll not go into detail, but his obsessions involved a fascination with women who were both obese and naturally blond. He could look at a blond across the room and instantly tell you whether the hair color came out of a bottle. We were dealing with strong issues, of false guilt and true guilt and other complexities. A secondary matter was the several excruciating migraines he suffered monthly. His physician in desperation had him on narcotics, trying to stabilize both his headaches and his erratic behavior.

When I took him off the narcotics, a necessary first step in order to introduce other therapy, he climbed the walls. We put him on Taradol to control his headaches. Only after we intervened with the Taradol and thereby reduced his distracting migraines could we work on issues. In Michael's case, a warm bath and some tension relief obviously would not have done it.

In another case, a couple came for marital help. Both of them suffered severe migraines, though that's not why they came. They came to find a solution to their violent fights. The husband's headaches were being managed with Sumatriptan, but the wife was taking a whole fistful of medications, trying to curb her unmanageable migraines. In order to work on her marriage problems, I pulled her off all that medication and put her on an antidepressant, which also has antipain components. She did great. Relieved at last, she could work on the hard knots of life.

Incidentally, the one-two combination of analgesic and antidepressant can work in two ways because fifty percent of migraineurs are also depressed. It's extremely common.

Certainly, medicines have their down sides, their side effects. Some are addicting; we have to be very careful with their use. But if you really need a narcotic, I won't hesitate to prescribe it.

The best known medications are detailed in chapter five and mentioned in chapter seven.

Be advised that medication is never a substitute for prevention, home remedy, and diet. Do your best to employ those first three steps to the maximum. If you need it, then, medication becomes an addition to those three pursuits. And if you do require medication, take it even as you continue pursuing the first three steps. They will help your medication do its job better.

On from Here

These four steps are your first steps toward managing headaches. They will help you in the immediate task of bringing the misery under control. But they are not the end. They are the beginning. The end is to diminish the intensity and frequency of your headaches permanently.

As we go on from here to explore the other three prongs of the seven-pronged cure, you may encounter a stumbling block. It will be a sense of despair. Is it worth all this?

The answer, of course, is, "Absolutely!"

You see, back at the very beginning, I reminded you that headaches are not a disease. They are only a symptom. Something else is wrong. That means something else is crying to be improved or put to rights. That is what we will do next.

CHAPTER 15

The Seven-Pronged Cure, Part II: Mind and Spirit

When Alicia was maybe seven or eight months old, she would take wonderful delight in simple things, as babies do. "Dance" a particular doll around while making funny noises, and she'd roll in the aisles. Of course, her infectious laughter immediately got everyone else rolling in the aisles as well.

A part of her expression of joy was clapping her hands.

Clapping hands. Why do banquet goers clap for the speaker before he or she has spoken? They don't have anything to applaud yet. The gesture is a welcome, a sign of gladness the world over, a statement that "we're so happy you're here!" And of course, if the speaker excels and really touches hearts, quite likely the audience will not only clap enthusiastically at the end of the speech but might even stand up to do it.

A standing ovation. Does it touch the speaker? You better believe it! Clapping? Absolutely! Many performers claim they work for that applause, that approval. Not the money, not even the power. The applause. And it all goes back to a little baby clapping.

Do you know how to make a baby happier? Physically take its hands in yours and clap them (gently, of course!). You see, clapping, a response to pleasure, works in the other direction as well. The act of clapping promotes pleasure. In chemistry you would call that a reversible reaction. The chemical change can go from A to B or from B to A. This reversibility of human actions and reactions lies at the heart of the final three prongs of headache management.

5. Insight into Personality and Feelings

A lasting cure for headaches begins with the immediate steps we discussed in chapter fourteen, the first four prongs of our seven-pronged attack. Understanding your innermost feelings and motivations is the next prong.

How important is insight into yourself? I'm thinking now of a seminary student I knew, a young woman. She had migraine for years. Years! She tried all sorts of medications, saw internists, took one psychological test after the other. They were looking for sources of stress, you see. Well, seminary is stressful, but she had the headaches before she enrolled. Then a friend—a mentor, actually—said, "You're angry with yourself, you've repressed it, and it has to vent somewhere. That's where the migraines are originating."

She was furious! She was absolutely certain he was misreading her. A month later she came to him and said, "I was so mad at you for saying that. I wasn't too mad to pray, though. God gave me insight; He could see whom I was angry with. Me. In two or three weeks, I was off medications and free of migraines."

Anger, anxiety, and stress all have to surface somehow. But people are very good at denying them, so good that they don't even know those things exist. That's why you can't stop with the first four steps of our attack. You have to go on to ferret out these hidden causes.

In Mark and Joan's case, we introduced these seven prongs over a period of weeks, the first order of business being to bring the headaches themselves under control. Now the hard work would begin, particularly for Joan.

This next step, insight, is important because every single person in the world has an underlying structure unique to himself or herself. Joan's deepest feelings and motivations were hers alone. And that underlying structure is what controls feelings, actions, and health.

Her situation was nothing at all like Mark's, though on the surface they shared many traits. On the other hand, another woman, Karen, also a migraineur, acted and thought exactly like Joan at the surface level, but her inner person, the power behind the conscious throne, differed profoundly.

Karen would never see forty again, but she was still a long way from fifty. Her dark hair showed only a few silver strands, and her supple body looked thirty. She exuded sweetness and light. No one who crossed her path failed to receive cheery greetings. She was the kind of relentlessly happy woman whom gossips would love to dump dirt about, except that Karen never did anything the gossips would find titillating.

Karen, like Joan, was a fireball of productivity. She served in her church as treasurer and president of the altar guild. In her local Christian Women's Club, she took her duties as book chairman so seriously that they averaged a hundred dollars a meeting in sales. For the Girl Scouts, she headed a Brownie troop, though her own daughter was in high school now. She was considered a paragon by all who worked with her. Her husband Gil was very proud of her; he said so to friends at church and work.

His greatest personal pride was that he had married—or trained, perhaps—the perfect Ephesians 5 wife, faultlessly obedient and caring. He never mentioned his sense of pride to Karen. It never occurred to him. She knew, and he knew she knew.

Now frequently as I delve into the subsurface dynamics of a person plagued with headaches, and particularly a migraineur, we find unresolved and displaced anxiety. In these cases, once the migraineur gets some insight into that anxiety, the headaches will usually wane or disappear altogether. Not always. I said usually.

In Karen's situation, to make a long case study short, her faultless obedience was doing her in. She was a woman with a mind of her own. Gil was a man with a mind of his own. Often the two minds did not match. But Karen was raised—trained, if you will, from early childhood—that the man's will prevails. She left "Love, honor, and obey" in her marriage vows. Gil directed every facet of her life. He determined whether she would take advantage of the eighteen-hour annual sale at the local department store, whether she would purchase a Whirlpool washing machine or a Kenmore. He even determined the length of her hair.

When we first talked about this, both Gil and she agreed that this was what they both wanted. She welcomed the control which relieved her of onerous responsibilities. She delighted in pleasing him. She wanted to make him happy. He in turn was demonstrating his love for her by caring about every detail. After getting all that out of the way, we dug down to her true feelings.

Karen was one smart woman, though she never consciously recognized that. But her native intelligence was being smothered by Gil's intense control. That hurt.

Down inside, as her exterior blithely smiled, she had to fight herself in order to obey her husband's whims and edicts. Defiance flared when she considered them unfair or overly restrictive (even at an unconscious level). She had to beat that defiance down as well as the anger which perceived unfairness always generates. On top of that she was angry with herself for "spinelessly obeying" (her words, as we intensively probed and talked about it).

I find this dichotomy constantly in frustrated, angry, anxiety-laden people of either sex. The person under control is torn by obedience versus defiance. When obedience wins, the person is angry for knuckling under. When defiance wins, the person is angry for not being more cooperative. In either case the anger seems inappropriate, so the person quashes it. Resentment results from having to bury the intense emotions.

The controller is in no better shape. Overcontrol provides no real satisfaction and certainly no happiness, despite all the controllee's efforts to keep the controller happy. It leads instead to even greater overcontrol as the controller frantically tries to maintain a grip on something he or she cannot really control at all. A constant undercurrent of fear runs beneath the surface of the controller—a fear that the grip will be lost.

Those were the true inner feelings in Karen and Gil's case. They were not present in Joan and Mark. Although on the surface Joan and Karen were both unremittingly cheery and productive, their appearances arose out of very different dynamics.

Joan was not overcontrolled. In fact, Mark and Joan's effects on each others' lives was quite evenhanded and mutual. They both vented anger and other feelings in healthy ways. When I went probing, I found no significant anger. What I found was fear.

Joan had grown up in a home where she was expected to succeed in any endeavor she attempted. Oh, her parents never said out loud, "Now we expect you to get all A's, Joan, and achieve the highest rank in Girl Scouts that there is." The expectation was assumed. Not even implied. Assumed. Joan would succeed. Period.

From the very beginning, her whole sense of worth was based solidly on her observed achievements. What she did defined who she was. And it had better be top-notch. Beneath the surface, below conscious level, Joan relentlessly feared goofing up somewhere, somehow, and thereby losing all worth and significance as a person.

Joan vehemently denied that. She insisted she was loved. True. She was valued. True. She enjoyed everyone's approval, and that's the sign of a good person. False. No honest person can please everyone. Joan tried so hard to accomplish the impossible and feared failure of any sort so much that the unbearable stress was causing physical illness—specifically, migraine.

Joan and Karen had the advantage of professional counsel to reach their feelings below conscious level. You may want to consider that yourself. If you're a migraineur, you might have to do so. However, if professional help is not a practical option at this time, try some of the following exercises to put this fifth prong into effect. Better by far, though, is to do the exercises with a trusted friend, swapping answers and insights. The two of you can hear and see things in each other that you'd miss in yourselves. Both of you will profit. And if you can possibly do so, handle all this with a lot of prayer.

Getting Past the Surface of Self

First, list ten words off the top of your head, no pausing or pondering, that describe your spouse, if you have one. If you do not, describe a close friend of the opposite sex. Set that list aside.

Similarly, write down ten words that describe you. Put that list aside also.

Do so now before you read further.

Now consider these next questions as essay-type questions to be thought about, discussed, explored. Spend plenty of time on them so that you can see beyond your surface.

1. What is your early training?

• When you were growing up, what was the observed relationship between Mom and Dad? Recall details and scenes.

- Analyze what you learned in school about man-woman relationships.
- What did you learn about those relationships at church? Exactly what did your church (from Sunday school or the pulpit) teach about men's and women's worth, responsibilities, and roles when you were growing up?
- List ten words to describe the perfect person whom the world needs.
- What is your attitude today toward the sexes? List ten words off the top of your head that describe each sex in general ways.

Compare those lists with the ones you built about you and your spouse. How do they differ? Now discuss, with a trusted person if possible, or with yourself alone if you must, how the shaping influences of early years are influencing your attitudes today. Spend time on this, lots of time. Spend prayer, too, if you can. Look at the lists often and analyze what they say between the lines. If you amend them, save the originals.

The lists will provide insight into what you really think; that is their purpose. For example, do your spouse and/or parents approach your ideal? Exceed the ideal? Do you suppose the spouse really is like that, or are you whitening or blackening the picture, based on your upbringing?

2. What are your attitudes today?

Think about the following traits and look for them in yourself, delving as deeply as you can into experiences you remember, phrases that stick in your memory, even the relative positions of people in group pictures. Try to place yourself outside yourself, so to speak, and go at it as if you were a detective assigned to investigate you.

Not all of these phrases will describe you, but some of them will. Check the ones that apply to you.

- Hiding limitations; you try to appear strong, even superhuman
- Hiding emotions from others; also from self
- Overly controlling, including control of emotions
- Afraid of warm feelings; keep people at distance
- Live for tomorrow, postpone pleasure
- Focus overly on details
- Strong willed, stubborn
- Exaggerated expectations for self
- Chronic worrier
- Driven, rigid, perfectionistic
- Need approval of everyone significant in your life
- Perfection is a worthy goal, whether obtainable or not
- You see success as equally worthy
- Believe seeking help equals admitting defeat
- Believe a human being's worth depends upon achievement of some sort (In other words, murdering a medical doctor would be a greater crime than murdering a street derelict.)

In these exercises you've looked at yourself. Now think about your relationships with other people.

Sorting out Relationships

1. What are the interpersonal dynamics between you and the people closest to you?

To explore this one, become a television producer. Pretend that you are going to prepare a miniseries about your life and relationships. You've been shooting the footage your whole life, recording all the details. But an awful lot of that is deadly boring—waiting in line at the checkout, getting the oil changed, mowing the lawn, sleeping, nodding off during endless business meetings at work as some fellow worker drones on and on. You're going to have to edit heavily. But edit what?

First, list by name the significant others in your life: parents, stepparents, grandparents, siblings, spouse(s), kids, close friends, relatives including deceased and absent.

To retain what is important and delete what is of limited use, examine your relationship with each of those significant other persons in turn, exploring these points as they apply to that person (sift carefully through the tapes of the past):

- How closely you listen when they talk
- How well you anticipate their needs and preferences
- How comfortably you obey or are obeyed
- How much you depend upon their acts and accomplishments
- How you feel when they are near
- How you feel when they leave
- What you like about them
- What you want to change about them
- What things in your life would improve if they were suddenly to die (or if they have already died)

Joan and Karen both were frightened at first to think about that last item as it pertained to their husbands. That's natural. But it cuts past the grief issues we immediately associate with a death and reveals much about faults in the relationship. The grief process, at least at first, puts the deceased on a pedestal. You want to find the real relationship.

Putting It Together

After all this has been considered, put together a documentary of your relationships. To do so honestly, you will have to incorporate what you determined about yourself in the first part of this extensive exercise. Those qualities strongly influence your relationships. In turn, the relationships through the years shape a great deal of your inner structure. Mutual influence.

Joan wagged her head. "Do you realize how little I've really done all these years? The same things over and over. A comfortable rut. And Mark and I both applauded them because I looked busy."

Karen was aghast for other reasons. "My husband controls me. My dad did. My aunt did. Even my teenagers do—not up front, because they're tightly disciplined. Gil keeps a close lid on their behavior. They do it by manipulation. I've been striving so long to stay nice to everyone, I've never ever been my own person."

What has all this to do with headaches, and how do we use it? We have arrived at the sixth prong.

6. Cognitive Restructuring

Joan was getting antsy. Her time of the month was approaching, and with it the prospect of another killer headache. We were pretty sure we had her immediate problem under control and the month would pass headache-free, but she couldn't help worrying. "If I quickly work through these prongs of yours," she asked, "do you suppose I can be done and well before headache time gets here? You know what I mean?"

"Yes and no. Yes, I know what you mean, and no, working through the prongs, as you call it, won't cure you instantly because it is an ongoing process. But we should see excellent results. You now have a good grasp of what's going on deep inside you. That's the essential first step to long-term relief."

The traits itemized in question two can all, to a greater or lesser extent, warp relationships and generate either overcontrolling or overly passive responses to others. I have found that headache sufferers, migraineurs in particular, usually display several of these characteristics prominently.

Beyond Logic

Your head and heart are two different beasts, running on different tracks ("Oh, don't I know!" moaned Karen). Cognitive recognition—that is, the head's understanding—is therefore not enough. Until the heart comes around, you'll slip right back into the headache-generating ways of doing and thinking, because ultimately, the heart controls.

But the head is an essential first step. Initially you get the head thinking in new ways. You restructure what your head "knows" by seeing what it is doing now (the purpose of prong 5) and then changing that. As a second step, and remembering that the heart is still functioning in the old ways, you alter your behavior to fit the new ways. Through changing the head's thoughts and the body's behavior, you will with time alter the heart's direction.

Here are the baby's hands being clapped, do you see? You generate happiness in the baby by physically performing the actions the baby performs when he or she is happy. That response is on a primal level. We're taking it to an infinitely deeper level. But the principle is the same.

The new you, having recognized stressful situations and relationships, will be able to deal with them constructively. You will no longer need an unrecognized, unspoken outlet for anger, fear, frustration, and anxiety. Usually, good-bye headaches.

Headaches aside, see how much healthier you will be!

So do headaches happen only to people who are sick in the head somehow? Not at all. Usually, there are only isolated areas in life where a person needs to pay attention, perhaps one or two of what might be called bad messages, derived from life, that the heart dwells upon. The two biggest:

"I must be perfect," and "I must have everyone's love and approval, God's approval, that certain someone's approval." Oh, the people who hurt us unwittingly, simply by not loving us enough!

What do others say?

"Nothing is more costly, nothing is more sterile, than vengeance."
—Winston Churchill

"Darkness cannot drive out darkness; only light can do that. Hate cannot drive out hate; only love can do that."
—Martin Luther King, Jr.

As a guide to your new thinking, let me take each of the items in your self-assessment questionnaire and recast them as positive statements. These are the statements you should make into solid head knowledge. They reflect the reality of life and of your needs.

"Now wait a minute." Joan raised a hand. "I've heard all this a hundred times."

"Certainly you have. But we're looking at all this from the standpoint of headache management. As a part of that management, you have to consider these matters anew. Call it a reminder."

Focus on these statements, reprogramming your thinking where you need to:

- Trying to appear strong and denying limitations very often causes headache. Since it serves no purpose and undermines health, present a more realistic, true-to-yourself pose to the world.
- Let others see your emotions and know what you feel. Learn to verbalize what you think. I've learned that tact is required but lying is not. This saying what I feel is a very personal point with me, and I can see many times in my life where it has held me in good stead.
- Control what you can and ought to control, and let the rest be.
- Warm feelings are as valuable as logic.
- In the end, all that will count is people.
- You may partake of good things now as well as tomorrow.
- Never lose the broad, overall picture.
- Learn when to bend, as a favor to someone if for no other reason.

- You're human. It's okay to goof up.
- Worry only about those things that you can change or improve by worrying.
- Lighten up.
- You will never obtain the approval of everyone significant in your life. Set standards and boundaries that are yours and maintain them.
- Perfection and success are worthy secondary goals; the primary goal is maturity and growth. You want to be mature, not perfect.
- It's nice to succeed, but it's not essential in every little endeavor.
- Every craftsman, technician, and scientist in his or her field of expertise depends upon the special skills of others. Seeking help equals being smart.
- Every human being's worth is intrinsic. No externals need to be considered.

Karen studied the list. "These involve emotions. Even I know logic won't resolve emotions."

"Many of the points in that list aren't logical," I answered.

"Take 'It's okay to goof up.' Not logical. Realistic, taking into account human frailty, but not logical. I've gone beyond logic with this, to plain observation and knowledge of the human condition."

The human condition includes grieving. Grieve what? Pain. Lost time, lost relationships, lost feelings that evaporated because of the headaches. Joan had her illness and its attendant problems to grieve; Karen needed to grieve the happiness lost to buried resentments.

What in your life did you lose because of your headaches and their underlying causes?

The list above itemizes messages you should be pounding into your conscious. Not all of them will apply to your situation as revealed by your insight-seeking. In fact, most of them will not. But you need desperately those that do. Repeat the relevant ones. Meditate upon them. Affix them in your mind.

The Message Bombardment

By far the best way to overcome the majority of headaches is to maintain a tranquil mind. By far the best way to do that is to immerse yourself in Scripture. You are constantly being pummeled by messages from all directions, with all sorts of agendas behind them. Those messages all shape us—we never truly forget anything we ever hear. Peace comes of knowing God and His will, and that comes from His Word.

Karen was very receptive to the voice of God through Scripture. She took to heart Psalm 34, especially verse 4: "I sought the LORD, and He heard me, and delivered me from all my fears." Psalm 56:3 was hard to apply, because she was often unaware that she was afraid. It had to be applied to deep-down fears, not surface stuff. That's always difficult. But it was do-able for Karen and it's do-able for you.

For the sake of people who, like Joan, are not heavily into Scripture-based truth, I have not detailed each of the aforementioned positive statements with Scripture quotations. Rest assured, each item in the list is scripturally sound. Every human being, for example, has intrinsic worth. God says so. He reveals that He knew us while we were as yet unborn.

It's not enough for me to casually suggest turning to the Bible for healing. Let me suggest some specific ways to do that.

One way is to devote time each day to simply reading the Bible, pausing at every chapter to think about what you just read. Another might be to spend time in meditation with a good devotional book such as *My Utmost for His Highest,* the Oswald Chambers classic. Still another is to use a book such as *100 Ways to Live a Happy and Successful Life,* by Paul Meier, States Skipper, and myself, or *100 Ways to Obtain Peace.*

Joan made this telling statement some months into her treatment: "I know now that if you continue with negative thinking, it produces headaches all by itself. And I can see how my thinking has slowly changed. But I can't tell what my heart is doing. What about the attitudes below my conscious thinking?"

7. New Behavior

Here is the prong that for Joan and for you will drive conscious attitudes down to where they will do some good. Make your behavior match your new convictions whether the heart goes along at first or not. Get that baby clapping!

Is it powerful? Let me tell you a story.

Helen handled these three steps splendidly. She gained insight, did her homework, and made a fine job of her cognitive restructuring, then launched out into new behaviors. Out of the blue, her father divorced her stepmother (her birth mother had divorced him), and he came out to stay with her a few months.

The guy was a jerk—neglectful, an adulterer (with both wives), a wastrel. Throughout her life, Helen had been trying in vain to earn his love. Within days she was back to stuffing her feelings, trying to please him, trying to make it all right this time around. She withdrew, suffered migraines every day, developed agoraphobia, and ended up taking all sorts of medications. She spent six years in her bedroom. When her father finally got tired of hanging around her house and went off to marry his third wife, she was suicidal. Back to steps five through seven!

Helen figured out anew how to find and vent her fierce anger. That discovery came with intense counseling in a hospital setting. She had to learn to forgive. That took some doing. Finally, she got back to this step and learned new behavior in order to bring her heart to where it had to be if she were to return to a functional life. In six weeks she was over her panic attacks and headaches, the agoraphobia, and the de facto loss of her father figure. Helen was able to get through life capably with very little medication. A few months after leaving the hospital, she could handle life without any medication. It took her six months to learn how to handle her problems, six years to wallow in regression, another six weeks to relearn it all, and six months to learn not to regress.

Yes, learning and practicing new behavior works. But it's not a simple one-shot cure.

Joan didn't have nearly as hard a time as Helen. She didn't progress down her rocky road as quickly as Helen did, but then, her road wasn't nearly as rocky. She decided she had to declare as her own the verse in Peter, "[God] cares for you." She had to change her heart from "You are only as good as your next accomplishment" to "You have value. Period. You do not have to kill yourself measuring up."

She did that in several ways. One technique was to reduce her activities and responsibilities and use the time to either further her own growth or simply do something nice for herself once.

Joan said, "I was always so busy I never had time for what I wanted to do. I can't even remember in childhood having any unstructured goof-off time. I don't know how to play. I have to take lessons on how to have a good time. The guilt is what I have to fight most. It seems selfish, giving up outside activities to make time for myself. Delicious and sinful and selfish and . . . and . . . it feels so good!"

Karen says, "Guilt. Oh, my yes. I was the church treasurer for eighteen years, and I hate bookkeeping. All the time, I felt intensely guilty for not liking the job or wanting to do it, since they needed a treasurer. And if I'd said no I would have felt even guiltier for letting them down somehow.

"Three months ago I turned in my resignation. Our pastor panicked. He absolutely panicked. 'But Karen, you're the only one who knows the books!' Of course I was the only one who knew the books. I'd been doing it through four different pastors. 'We can't find anyone else who will do it,' he said.

"I answered him with, 'I'm giving sixty days' notice. If you can't find one in sixty days, I guess you'll have to go without.' I couldn't believe I said that. It sounded so cruel. Cold. But as I said it, the strangest feeling came over me, as if a load of bricks had just dropped off my shoulders. Really! It was that vivid. Anyway, they found a retired lady who said she'd do it. But if they hadn't, I think I could have stood firm. Forty-three years old, and I'm finally able to set some decent boundaries."

Why did these women abandon their obligations?

The answer is they did not. Both paid their dues, serving long and well. Both had given ably. They were not letting someone down or ducking out of performing service. They had paid by their gifts, energies, and time and also by putting aside their own needs and desires in order to serve others. Yet their needs were as definite and as valuable as anyone else's.

The reason they put aside some of these tasks, for Joan especially, was to reinforce the new head knowledge that their worth was intrinsic and not based upon accomplishment. Within a year they were taking on new tasks, but with a difference. Now they were judicious, learning by painful degrees to say no to some requests, and taking jobs that interested them. For once, their gifts gave them personal satisfaction and fun.

For example, since childhood Joan had always wanted to own a horse. Her parents had said no. When she grew up she never had time. These days, she's a volunteer wrangler at a handicapped kids' camp.

She hasn't had a migraine in fourteen months.

Your New Behavior

Having gained some insight into yourself, what have you found? Think about that. Now think about what you might do—physical action, we're talking about here—to firm up those insights. You want your body actions to feed back into your heart.

Is anxiety a problem for you? When you start to get anxious, immediately take a deep breath.

Stop and consider that simple action—merely taking a breath. Let's say one of my girls is going to buck a fifty-pound bag of chicken mash. Without even thinking about what she's doing, she takes a deep breath and holds it while she heaves the sack up into the back of the Jeep. Then she resumes breathing normally. When you are about to heft a heavy weight, you do that, too. Our actions control our breathing, and to an amazing extent our breathing controls our actions. When you suck in a deep breath you're ready for something. You can feel it.

Feelings of anxiety for you must be a signal to relax. Your altered behavior then alters the tension.

Mark's problem was tension, so he deliberately injected more humor into his life. He sought out the company of loony friends who could make him laugh. You probably know a couple such people yourself. You see, laughter releases as much tension as does crying. Mark was raised to believe that men don't show their emotions. For him, laughing was much more acceptable than crying.

Tailor your means of release similarly. But find a release. I love this quote of Norman Vincent Peale: "Americans are so tense and keyed up that it is impossible even to put them to sleep with a sermon."

A

Pain—Its Causes and Its Cures

Headaches. They're not all the same. They can be mild or severe, dull or sharp, acute to chronic, short to long. They come at different times for different reasons. You've probably suffered from one or more of these types of headaches:

Tension Headaches

- Can be chronic; steady pressure or pain.
- Worse during times of stress.
- Usually located in the front and/or back of the head (bilateral).
- Constant band-like pressure lasting for hours or days.
- May be worse at the end of the day.
- May recur regularly for weeks, months, or years.
- Most common of all headaches.
- Usually begins after the age of ten.
- Muscles tighten in the face, neck, shoulders, or jaws.

- Sufferer can continue to function.
- Common causes: standing in long lines, conflict, taking a test, driving in heavy traffic, noisy environment, etc.

Migraine Headaches

- Throbbing or pulsating severe pain.
- Frequently just on one side of the head (unilateral) but can be bilateral or switch sides.
- Often accompanied by nausea and vomiting.
- Recurs at irregular intervals (days, months, years).
- Builds over minutes to hours to a steady pain that persists for two to twenty-four hours.
- Pain tends to be around the eyes.
- Can be incapacitating to the point that the person can't function in normal routines.
- Tends to be hereditary (60 to 70 percent of the cases).
- Some have neurological effects such as weakness of an arm or leg.
- Related to vessel constriction and dilation.
- A quiet, dark environment can speed recovery.
- Afflicts women three times more often than men.
- Often begins in one's twenties and fades in the forties.
- Seeking medical attention is important.
- Lifestyle may trigger migraines: skipping meals, becoming stressed or fatigued, exercise, smoking, or sleeping late.
- More frequent in perfectionistic, compulsive personalities.
- Certain foods containing chemical substances may trigger migraines in some people.

- Other triggers are allergies, air pressure changes, and pollutants.
- Classic migraines are usually preceded by an aura (visual disturbances) where the visual field is reduced or there may be flashing lights that look like starbursts or wavy lines.

Cluster Headaches

- Occur in clusters of short duration, usually without warning (as often as twelve to fifteen times a day for periods up to ninety minutes).
- Pain is on one side of the head (unilateral), usually behind the eye.
- Pain is severe and steady (the most excruciating of all headaches); often occur at night.
- May disturb vision and involve nasal congestion and tearing.
- May be triggered by alcohol, smoking, specific foods, stress, or glare.
- Often no family history.
- Predominantly in middle-aged men (ages thirty to fifty).
- Pain begins abruptly, lasting less than two hours (and may occur daily at the same time).
- Clusters come in bouts of days to weeks and recur at intervals for months to years; remissions can last a year or more.
- Seek medical attention.
- Clusters tend to be more common in the spring and fall; there may be a link to histamine.

Headaches of Head Trauma

- Constant dull ache with superimposed throbbing.
- Usually within a day of injury to the head.
- May be localized.
- Associated problems: trouble with memory, concentration, emotional instability, irritability, equilibrium.

Headaches Asociated with Vascular Disorders

- Anoxia, aneurysm, hemorrhage, hypertension, vasculitis, stroke, visual malformation, lupus, temporal arteritis, basilar artery, and others.

Headaches Associated with Nonvascular Disorders (Rare)

- Meningitis, brain tumor, cyst, abscess, subdural hematoma.
- Worse with excessive coughing, changing head position; double vision.
- Usually accompanied by other neurologic symptoms (loss of coordination or strengths) because of the increased intracranial pressure.
- Seek medical attention.

Headaches Associated with Chemical Substances or Their Withdrawal

- Excessive use of alcohol; hangover headache may relate to the alcohol's affect of dilating vessels, histamine release, or breakdown products of the alcohol.
- Food allergy headaches.

- Caffeine withdrawal (common).
- Birth-control pill headaches.

Headaches Associated with Systemic Infection

- Examples: syphillis, tuberculosis, fungal infections, sarcoidosis, herpes.
- Almost any disease that can cause fever.

Headaches Associated with Metabolic Abnormality

- Hypoglycemia (low blood sugar); in such cases, the previous meal may not have provided enough protein, carbohydrates, and/or fats to maintain normal blood-sugar levels. Eating healthy between-meal snacks may help.
- Hunger headache.

Pain Associated with Diseases of the Head and Neck

- Eye disorders, glaucoma, refractory error (consult an eye doctor).
- Arthritis of the cervical spine.
- Lesions of the teeth, tongue, ear, or throat.
- Jaw joint dysfunction (clicking or popping noise, bilateral pain, limited movement, tenderness).

OTHER HEADACHES

While all headaches could be placed under the above headings of the new International Classifications, breaking out the following types might be helpful.

Trigeminal Neuralgia

- Pain above the temporal area (temples) usually in older people. The sedimentation rate is high, and they respond to Tegretol.
- More common in women.
- Burning and aching in the temples.

Hypertension Headaches

- Traditionally thought to occur upon awakening (which they can) but can occur at other times as well.
- Most hypertension (high blood pressure) has no symptoms at all; that's why it's known as the "silent killer." However, if the blood pressure is extremely high (over 180 systolic and over 100 diastolic), headache pain may be present.

Cough Headaches

- Distinctive, brief, severe, bursting after a cough.
- Often in middle-aged men.

Lumbar Puncture Headaches *(Spinal Tap)*

- Self-limited.
- Many who have had lumbar (back) punctures can attest to this pain.

Allergy or Sinus Headaches

- Allergies from pollens, dust, feathers, animal hair, or foods can cause headache pain. Skin tests are helpful in determining specific allergies.
- Common cause: allergic rhinitis or hay fever.
- Common organic headaches are caused by acute sinus infection (blocked sinus drainage resulting from colds, allergies, or bacterial infections).

Toxic Headaches

- Countless chemicals can cause headaches.
- Exogenous—chemicals originating from without the body, such as pesticides, preservatives, smog, polluted water, insecticides, fuels, paint, cleaning fluids.
- Endogenous—chemicals originating within the body, such as viral, bacterial, rickettsial (can be severe).

Sex or Exercise Headaches

- Rare, painful.
- May be related to excitement, increased blood pressure or heart rate.

Postseizure Headaches

- Headaches often occur after a grand mal seisure.

Because of possible side-effects and other concerns, use medication with great caution and discernment. Used ineffectively, medicine will not produce the desired results. Used inappropriately, the medicines are dangerous. Not considered at all, excellent science is for nought.

The medical treatments for headaches fall into several categories. Non-narcotic pain relief medicine has been around since ancient times. The Romans, Greeks, and American Indians used the bark of the willow tree for pain relief.

Aspirin (or salicylate, which is found in many trees and other plants) has sold more than any drug in history. (Forty billion aspirins are consumed each year in America.) Coated aspirin are designed to cause less stomach irritation but may be less effective due to decreased absorption. Aspirin, like other medicines, can have significant side-effects (ulcers, ringing in ears, Reye's Syndrome in children, poisoning, etc.). However, aspirin has generally proven safe for most people and is often the first choice for management of mild to moderate headaches.

Tylenol® and nonsteroidal antiinflammatory drugs (NSAIDS), including Advil® and Motrin® (ibuprofens), Anaprox®, Naprosyn®, Feldene®, Clinoril®, Tolectin®, Orudius®, Nalfon®, Indocin®, Voltaren®, and Meclomen® have also been used extensively. These can have side-effects such as stomach irritation.

Narcotic pain medicines (codeine, morphine, Demerol®, Talwin®, Percodan®, Vicodin®) have also been prescribed. They can be extremely effective but unfortunately are addicting and can produce a dependency. They are used with great caution by most doctors today, especially for chronic headaches, as they can actually increase the pain through a phenomenon called rebound and withdrawal state. I rarely prescribe any controlled narcotic medicines for the pain.

Ergotamine (Gynergen®, Bellergal®), like caffeine (Cafergot® is caffeine plus ergotamine), is a vasoconstrictive agent that has brought relief to many individuals with migraine headaches. It should be used only to abort acute attacks. While it is not addicting, it (along with caffeine) is one of the most often abused drugs by people with chronic headaches. Used regularly it exacerbates their condition, causing withdrawal headaches. Midrin®, a drug similar to ergotamine, has successfully been used to abort and prevent mixed headaches. It is probably less effective than ergotamine but may have fewer side-effects.

Antidepressants (Elavil®, Tofranil®, Sinequan®, and Norpramin®) have been used with excellent results in reducing the intensity and frequency of pain in some individuals with chronic headaches. Low doses actually treat the underlying serotonin factors.

Beta blockers such as propranolol or Inderal® are used to help prevent vascular headaches. But don't use them if you have certain heart problems, diabetes, asthma, or are pregnant.

Prednisone is sometimes prescribed for cluster headaches.

Minor tranquilizers (Serax®, Librium®, Klonopin®, etc.) may relieve tension and muscle strain and decrease headaches. Sansert® has been used to prevent migraines but serious side-effects are possible. Periactic®, an antihistamine, has been used for headaches but can cause drowsiness and should not be used in the presence of glaucoma or urinary retention.

Major tranquilizers (Thorazine®, Mellaril®) have

been used but are often not appropriate for the mere relief of headache pain. Lithium has been used for cluster headaches. Anticonvulsants (Dilantin®) have been used for migraine. Calcium channel blockers (Calan®, Isoptin®) have also been used for migraine prevention. Tegretol® has been used for a rare form of headaches—trigeminal neuralgia.

Diuretics have been used for migraines associated with the menstrual cycle. Though not approved for such, Catapres® and monamine oxidase inhibitors have been used to treat migraines.

Imitrex® is a very effective new medication. Ask your doctor about it.

Note: Consult your physician before taking any of these medicines. Side-effects may be dangerous for some people.

Index

About the Author

Dr. Frank Minirth is a diplomate of the American Board of Psychiatry and Neurology and received an M.D. degree from the University of Arkansas College of Medicine. He is cofounder of the Minirth Meier New Life Clinics and has coauthored more than 30 books, including *Love Is a Choice, Love Hunger, The Father Book, Things That Go Bump in the Night, The Anger Workbook, The Path to Serenity, Worry-Free Living, Happiness Is a Choice,* and *You Can.*

Dr. Minirth resides in Plano, Texas with his wife and five daughters.